Alzheimer's and the Workplace

A communication guide for anyone who encounters Alzheimer's

Alzheimer's
and
the Workplace

A communication guide for anyone who encounters Alzheimer's

Patricia M. Thompson

St. Colman Press

P.O. Box 17634

Rochester, NY 14617

ISBN: 1-4116-3037-8
Library of Congress Control Number: 2005901427

Published by

St. Colman Press
P.O. Box
Rochester, NY 14617

In conjunction with

Lulu Enterprises
3131 RDU Center, Suite 210
Morrisville, NC 27560

Lulu ID #: 122998

This book is dedicated to my aunt, Mary Manion, who, in 1978, took the first tentative steps with me on the road of Alzheimer's Disease.

And to my daughter, Michelle Dawson, who, in 2000, encouraged me to take much bolder steps and start my teaching business, St. Colman Consulting.

TABLE OF CONTENTS

Preface

This book has been written for all caregivers, both personal and professional, full-time and occasional, who would like to find a way to communicate more effectively with people who have dementing illnesses. Personal experience led me to learn these skills and, eventually, to share them with others through St. Colman Consulting, my teaching business.

In 1987, we began to recognize problems in my Mother's behavior and memory. We found ourselves in the role of long-distance caregivers, myself in New York, and Mom in New Mexico, my sisters in Arizona. In 1989, with a confirmed diagnosis of Alzheimer's Disease, she came to live with me. I had a few years' exposure to this disease by that time as I had two aunts with Alzheimer's whom I helped care for, but living with it 24 hours a day was something one cannot prepare for. In 1991, we moved Mom into a skilled nursing facility and a whole new perspective was gained. Now, after almost 20 years of caring for three family members with this disease, attending lectures, workshops and conferences, extensive reading and study, and spending numerous hours at nursing homes over the years (for personal reasons and as a volunteer with Hospice), I have learned a great deal about this illness and the people who have it. I have taken the various theories of care and communication and put them into practice, and I know what works and what doesn't. (I should qualify this by saying what works one day may not work the next; and what works with one person may not work with another. But there are a variety of options that can be tried). As a result, I have distilled the best of what I have learned and used, and I present it here.

If you can understand what makes a person tick, why he does the things he does, you can often find ways to reach him. There are two keys to reaching each individual: knowing who he was before this disease took over, and being able to go where he is now. These two points are vital to the type of communication skills I propose in this book and you will see them cropping up again and again. His personality, temperament, background, worklife, etc. will help you understand his actions, even though those actions are currently determined by his disease.

I have often heard it said that Alzheimer's causes a person's personality to change. However, it has been my observation that a person's basic personality doesn't change so much as it is exaggerated in inappropriate ways. For instance, my mother was always a fanatic about neatness and cleanliness. When she had Alzheimer's, she would do things like put garbage in an empty box and put it in the cupboard, or put dirty dishes in the cupboard. One day, after taking her out for ice cream, as I was going to drop some mail at the post office, she tried to get me to put her ice cream wrapper and napkin on the ground under the mailbox. Each of these incidents might cause you to say she would never have done any of these things before she had Alzheimer's. But consider that in each case, her objective was to get the troublesome, messy thing out of sight, to make things 'neat' again. She was unaware of the consequences of her actions, but her need to 'tidy up' came through with flying colors. When you know what type of personality the person had before the disease, you can, with a little imagination, anticipate some of the things he might or might not do. I'll offer more examples of this throughout the text.

Every Alzheimer's patient is someplace. More than likely, however, they are not in the same environment, day or time that you are. Neither one of you can see or experience where the other is, but you have the ability and imagination to go where he is and try to see what he sees; he cannot do the same. His is the environment in which you will communicate. When dealing with folks with dementia, you need to learn to occasionally throw reality out the window and get into his reality. Sometimes it's a fun trip.

Chapters I and II will be applicable to anyone who encounters someone with dementia, whether on an occasional basis, or a full-time personal or professional basis. The advice and suggestions in these chapters are tried and true methods. They can make your life and, more importantly, the life of the person in question, easier. While the information in these sections is often geared toward nursing home staff, home health aides or those who care for dementia patients in their work setting, it is equally applicable to any caregiver. The terminology, however, is written in terms of assisted living situations; residents, patients, group activities and so on.

Chapters III through VIII will address more specific topics and settings, but there is much to be gained in each of them for anyone who wants to know more about communication skills. For instance, Chapter VI is geared toward police and emergency workers, but applies equally to anyone who may encounter difficult or crisis behaviors from time to time and it goes hand in hand with Chapter III. There is a great deal of information about and for families and caregivers in Chapters IV, VII and VIII.

Chapter VIII goes in a somewhat different direction in that it looks at the effect of Alzheimer's Disease in the workplace setting – how does one recognize and deal with the employee with early stage Alzheimer's, how does the employer accommodate the employee-caregiver, and how does that employee-caregiver manage to give his or her best to both the job and the family member being cared for.

If the person you are caring for is someone close, a family member, I would like to make a recommendation that isn't necessarily easy to put into practice, but when you do, the benefits are great. As you progress through this disease with your loved one, the tendency is to keep looking back, to remember the person they were and the potential life they have lost. Consider, however, that this illness may go on for years and you will be wasting precious time wishing for what could have been.

What I would suggest is to take the memories of that person as he was and put them on a back burner, so to speak. If you want to draw any good out of this experience – and believe me, there is good as well as bad – you have to live where they are now. This is what you are dealing with now. This is real life, whether we like it or not. If you put the past away for safe keeping for now, it will still be there later when it's time to return and reclaim it.

When my mother had been in my care two or three years, I said to a friend, "I can't remember what she was like any more." I was feeling pretty sorry for myself because of it, but rather than just sympathizing with me, my friend said, "That's all right. You'll remember after she's gone." That was the best answer she could have given me. That's when it dawned on me that I needed to get on with life as it really existed. Once you can do that, you will start to experience 'golden moments.' There are joys to be had nearly every day that you would miss if you're spending all your time looking back and being sad. I've devoted all of Chapter IX to encouraging thoughts and some of these golden moments.

A final note: when I refer to "the nursing home" throughout the text, I am referring to the nursing home where my mother spent the last ten years of her life, Wesley Gardens. That is where the majority of my real life experience came from in dealing with dementia patients, my 'home away from home' for those ten years. I owe them a debt of gratitude for the loving care they gave my Mother during that sojourn.

Chapter I

Signs and Behaviors of Alzheimer's

One of the first things I am often asked is to define the difference between Alzheimer's and dementia. Dementia is an umbrella term that refers to symptoms of diminishing mental capacity. It is a loss of intellectual functioning (thinking, remembering, reasoning) which can be caused by any number of things, some of which are uncontrolled diabetes, adverse drug reaction, brain tumor, depression, and, of course, Alzheimer's Disease. Alzheimer's is the most prevalent cause of dementia.

The first person to recognize the onset of Alzheimer's is the person with the disease. Often it is not identified specifically as Alzheimer's, but the individual knows there is something wrong well before family and friends do. He may deny the existence of a problem and certainly, he can hide it for quite a while, but he knows. This is why when family and friends look back, they will often report that the first 'symptom' they noticed was the person's mood swings. Incidents of forgetfulness or feeling lost can cause fear and/or depression. "Good days" and "bad days" are more clearly defined in these early days and so a person's mood will often be a response to the type of day he is having. On good days, he feels as though perhaps it was all his imagination and surely, he is fine. On bad days, the fear and frustration comes back.

There are those who think the difference between normal memory problems and Alzheimer's is that with Alzheimer's you're not aware of your forgetfulness. This is not true. People with Alzheimer's do know they are having memory problems. They may not recognize it specifically as Alzheimer's, but they know it's something different than they have experienced before. They may deny it, they may try to hide it, but they do know. This is one of the main things that make this disease so sad in the earlier stages. When they are lucid, these folks know what is happening and where they are headed. I sometimes think it would be easier if they could step from a normal, clear-thinking world directly into that other world where they don't know what is happening to them any more.

So what is the difference between normal forgetfulness and Alzheimer's? If I forget where I put my keys, or forget a person's name or the details of an event that happened, eventually I will recall these things. Once I find the keys, I will recall putting them in that particular place. I may think of that person's name in the middle of the night, or bring back to mind the details of an event as I talk about it with someone. With Alzheimer's, however, once something is forgotten, it's as if that little piece of time is gone. It cannot be recovered. For instance, you are in a department store looking at items on the main floor. The next thing you are aware of, you are on the second floor and you have absolutely no recollection of having gone up an elevator, escalator or stairs. Those few moments of time are gone. You cannot bring them back to mind, nor will they occur to you later. This is because the loss of an incident in this case is the result of brain cells not 'firing' properly, not relaying the mental message. Normally, a message is relayed and stored, but 'mislaid.' Later on, you find it and "Oh yes, I remember putting the keys on the dining room table when I came in." In the case of Alzheimer's, the pathway of nerve cells was interrupted, the message was never stored in the first place; therefore, it cannot be recalled later.

"Normal aging forgetfulness is a result of the electrical system of the brain not firing efficiently and correctly all the time; information is not lost, but perhaps only temporarily unattainable. 'Mild Cognitive Impairment' is the result of a slowing down of the degradation of amyloid and may maintain a stable rate throughout an elder's life; some information is lost. Dementia is the result of little or no degradation of amyloid as it builds up in the brain."[1]

The progress of Alzheimer's can be broken down into several functional stages, but here I will just look at the general pattern and progress of this disease. Keep in mind that not all individuals will experience all of these effects, nor will they experience them in the same order. Also, it is difficult to qualify the various phases of Alzheimer's in terms of the length of time they will last. Alzheimer's can last from two to twenty years or more. So you can see that an initial stage could last a month or two in one person and a year or two in another. It has been my observation, although I don't know if this has been borne out in studies, that the younger one is when Alzheimer's takes hold, the more quickly the disease will progress. The progress of this disease can be thought of as a gradual downward slope with notable sudden drops following any traumatic episodes. Events such as a death in the family, a move, an emergency situation or even a large family gathering or a holiday can precipitate a noticeable regression. I didn't realize it at the time, but when we were planning for Mom's move into a nursing home, the people who did the review process for appropriate placement took this into consideration. While I felt she was operating at a level appropriate for one type of care, they evaluated her and recommended a more controlled care level, knowing that the move itself would cause a sudden decrease in abilities. This turned out to be true.

In the earliest phases of Alzheimer's, the person knows what is happening on some level or other. Initially, he can hide this from friends and family, but sooner or later, something different will be noticed. Some of the things reported as having been noticed first are fluctuation in mood, difficulty writing checks, handling money in a store, or taking phone messages. One might get lost in normally familiar surroundings or lose objects. Problem solving deficits may not be apparent unless the person is tested. When a person goes through a medical assessment, tests are performed to identify or eliminate all other possible causes of dementia. Some of these are correctable or at least treatable to the point of stopping further deterioration. When all other possibilities are eliminated, a diagnosis of Alzheimer's is presumed and testing becomes more a case of evaluating a person's current functional ability. Testing can include interviews and such things as having the person –

o   draw the face of a clock with a specific time

o   remember and repeat unrelated words

o   name parts of an object (band of a watch, brim of a hat)

o   give a list of words (name any animals/colors/foods you can think of)

o   demonstrate manual pantomime (show me how you would slice bread)

While there is no definitive physical test for Alzheimer's Disease, it has been studied and observed thoroughly enough that now the pattern of behaviors is fairly well defined.

Often, when a person appears and behaves quite normal most of the time, you won't notice his deficits until you converse at length with him or ask a slightly challenging question. Then the person's ability, or inability, to plan, organize or think abstractly will be seen. This is a very frustrating time for the individual because of others' reactions. First of all, if the person affected is very aware and willing to try to deal with this disease, he may have family members who are in denial and who refuse to acknowledge there is a problem. They may write it off to odd behavior or may attribute it to laziness, lack of concentration or unwillingness to cooperate. This only contributes to feelings of frustration and confusion on the part of the individual. On the other hand, once family members have recognized and accepted the illness, they may then assume the person is now incapable of handling anything for himself any more and they take away all responsibilities from him. Rev. Robert Davis, writing about his own experience of Alzheimer's, said, "…one mistake in my daily life will mean another freedom will be taken from me. One moment of inattention will change your life forever."[2] If you or I were to forget to turn off the oven, lock the door or pick up something at the store, it is just written off as a momentary lapse of memory. If an Alzheimer's person forgets something, it's assumed he cannot handle that particular responsibility any more. This is a very tentative line to walk for both the individual as well as his caregivers.

Medical caregivers – physicians, nurses, nursing home staff – can also be inadvertently guilty of insensitivity. They may expect too much of the impaired person, or they may not give him credit for the capabilities he does have. "Even the medical community has long assumed that people with Alzheimer's have little insight into their own impairments. As a result, they are treated in less than compassionate ways."[3] A gentleman in a support group was reported as having said, "Once people know I have Alzheimer's, I will never be treated the same again."

As time goes on, the person will experience something and then quickly forget the actual incident. Thoughts come into his mind and are gone. A sense of recollection is there, a remembrance of the feeling or emotion, but he can't define it or wrap words around it. For instance, one day my mother's caregiver, Debbie, and her two little children brought Mom home from an outing. The children stayed outside playing when Mom and Debbie came in. We just talked for a few minutes and Debbie left. All the while, Mom was standing in the front window stewing and grumbling and worrying about the children who had gone down the street a little ways. When Debbie left, Mom saw the little girl get in the car, but not the boy. She began to get frantic, thinking the child was lost. I reassured her that he was in the car and on his way home with his mother. She accepted that, but half an hour later, she started pacing, wringing her hands, and looking out the window. I asked her what was wrong, but she didn't know. I tried to remind her about the little boy and that he was safe, and once again, she calmed down. However, this behavior continued all evening long. After a couple rounds of it, she had no idea what I was talking about when I mentioned Danny and Debbie; she just knew she was supposed to be worried about something – and worry she did!

Another loss is being able to focus on or follow more than one thought or idea at a time. Things need to be broken down into individual steps. Once you get past two or more thoughts in one sentence, the person is lost. I had three aunts who lived together. One, Aunt Therese, had Alzheimer's. I was going over to take her out one day and I had called ahead to let Aunt Anne know I was coming. When I arrived, they were both frustrated nearly to the point of tears. Aunt Anne pleaded, "I can't get her to do anything! I told her you were coming to get her and take her to the lake for a concert and that she had better use the bathroom before you got here, but she won't go! She just stands there!" I told her not to worry, I'd take care of it. Then I turned and said, "Aunt Therese!" She looked at me. "Want to go out?" She nodded with a big smile. "Go to the bathroom." And she went right up. Give the person only one thing to digest at a time.

A person with Alzheimer's cannot plan complex tasks and often won't start anything on his own. Without the ability to think logically or in a step-wise manner, one cannot foresee a sequence of events or consequences of an action. There is no "if ... then" thinking. For instance, you cannot explain to the person with Alzheimer's that if he hides ice cream in the back of his closet, then it will melt. He only knows that he needs to keep it from someone *now* and save it for himself.

Suspicion and paranoia frequently come into play here. The person will accuse others of stealing things or accuse a spouse of cheating or hiding things. Two things contribute to this behavior. One is the lack of logic. You cannot reason with a person by saying that he is always putting his money in different places and it will be found as it has been in the past. He can't reason that out. There is no past. Nor can you say, 'No, I wasn't with someone else. I went to the store. See the groceries I bought?' There is no connection in his mind between the groceries and the fact that you had been gone for what seemed an eternity. There is a control issue at work here as well. As a person is gradually losing control over all aspects of his life – his work, his ability to drive, his ability to make decisions – he can't bear to face another loss. Therefore, if he cannot find his money or jewelry or whatever, it is easier to think that someone has stolen it rather than that he lost it. If someone took it, that is not his responsibility. But if he lost it, it's just one more thing that he has been 'irresponsible' about. Hiding and hoarding things go hand in hand with suspicion. Rev. Davis writes "...loss of self, the helplessness to control this insidious thief who was little by little taking away my most valued possession, my mind, had made me especially wary of the rest of my possessions in an unreasonable way."[2]

Another behavior that becomes evident at this point is the overwhelming need to do something or to go somewhere. Because the past and the future are fading, there is only now. And the lack of ability to understand sequence or consequence leads to the individual focusing on now. 'Now' turns out to be whatever is in his mind at the moment. If the notion occurs that he should go to Church, to the store, to work, whatever, that need becomes pressing. He will try his utmost to get there, and no logic will talk him out of it. This is where wandering begins. It's 2:00 a.m. and he's out of bed and out the door. You catch up to him and ask where he's going. "I have to go to the store." Typically, it will be "I have to…" "But," you say, "it's dark out. The store is closed." No it's not. The only reality in his mind right now is the store. He doesn't know that it's dark, or cold, or raining. When a person becomes this determined to do something, he becomes unaware of his environment.

Another worrisome feature of the mid-stages of Alzheimer's is the loss of self control and a sense of social graces. Because he is becoming unaware of his environment, he will often do whatever occurs to him to do at the moment. He may undress in public, walk into a busy street, bring strangers into the house. At one time, Mother was staying at my sister's house. My sister was at work and Mom couldn't figure out how to use the washing machine, so she went outside, found a man nearby (who, fortunately, turned out to be a gardener for the property) and brought him in to help her. People with Alzheimer's are often very trusting and unaware of danger. This can be an advantage when you are trying to help them or a disadvantage when they have wandered off on their own.

Restlessness occurs frequently in the evening. This is the well-known phenomenon of sun-downing. By late afternoon or early evening, people are tiring from their activities of the day and perhaps, of the struggle to hold the enemy, which is Alzheimer's, at bay. Somewhere in their subconscious there is a recollection of needing to come home from work, to fix dinner, to bring in the children from play, to finish up the day's activities and settle the family for the night. It all percolates into a restlessness or anxiety that is difficult to calm.

As social skills, and sequencing, and the ability to perform tasks are fading, the person now needs more assistance in choosing clothes, dressing, recalling day/date, telling time. However, he still can perform 'over-learned' behaviors when cued (handshake, putting in dentures, using silverware).

Unusual or difficult behavior can sometimes be the result of visual problems. Typically, a person with dementia will lose some degree of depth perception, nor can he pick out objects which are similar in color to the background. This type of misperception can result in the person becoming frightened or having physical accidents. Steps, furniture, doorways, even clothing or dishes, should have colors that contrast with the background so the individual can pick them out. In some rare instances, a person may only be able to see his right (or left) field of vision. If this is the case, and you walk or wheel him down a hallway, when you return, he will think he is in a completely different place.

As the person moves further into this disease, there is somewhat less stress. There is less awareness of personal loss in the mid to late stages. He is more out of touch with those around him. By this time, he has become disoriented with regard to time (day, night, hour of the day, seasons) and place (gets lost when he leaves home, disoriented within the home, wants to "go home" to a childhood home). Now he begins to become disoriented to people as well. From time to time, he may not recognize those closest to him or may think they are someone else. Before my mother lost the ability to speak, she would alternately call me by my name, by my sisters' names, by her sisters' names or she would call me Mother.

"Each minute of his life may consist of starting over with no memory of previous events. In this world, familiar objects disappear without explanation. The immediate environment, just moments ago filled with loved ones, now is populated only with strangers."[4]

Language abilities tend to regress in the following manner:

- normal conversational ability unless pressed into lengthy conversation or asked multiple questions
- able to convey thoughts and ideas; but sporadically substitutes incorrect words or stops for lack of ability to find right word
- still speaking in words and trying to convey thoughts; but without sensible construction
- combination of words and sounds; often repeats words or phrases over and over
- gibberish, few if any words; repeats sounds over and over
- little, if any, sounds; may make comfort or stressful sounds when content or uncomfortable

Hallucinations or delusions occur with some people. However, this is not harmful as long as it isn't frightening. More often than not, when he sees things we don't, he seems to think it's perfectly normal, not stressful at all. My aunt once looked out in the back entryway of their house and mistook some coats as St. Joachim and St. Anne. She only seemed disturbed because they wouldn't come in. We moved the coats. Another time, she was annoyed because there were "all these people in my bed at night. I hardly have room to sleep with all of them in there." She wasn't afraid, just annoyed. My mother once saw a face moving down the wall of our stairway. She thought it was quite lovely.

Another thing that may happen along the way is that he loses his sense of humor. More precisely, he cannot understand abstractions, sarcasm or double meanings. Since he tends to take things literally, he may not understand teasing. But this is not always the case. I have known people with dementia who have retained their sense of humor throughout their illness.

Demented patients are often described as being intensely focused or totally out of focus. One day my mother was tearing up a paper napkin into smaller and smaller pieces. I couldn't get her attention or distract her in any way. Just then a nurse dropped a metal tray right outside her door. I jumped three feet. Mom never blinked an eye, just kept tearing that napkin. So, on the one hand, you could say a person is out of focus; that is, you cannot direct their attention to what you want him to see or do. On the other hand, he is, indeed, totally focused. He becomes engrossed with what he wants to see or do and may become angry if you try to move him or change his focus.

Oftentimes a patient in these later stages, if he is still physically capable, wants to be on the move all the time. He rarely sits down and doesn't sleep for very long at a time. Eating may be a problem at this point if you can't get him to sit still for long or if he isn't aware that it is food in front of him. It turns out, however, that walking is good for Alzheimer's patients.

It is good for their physical health and the progression of the disease is slower than it is for those who just sit.

Eventually you start to see the breakdown of physical abilities. He cannot bathe himself, or handle the mechanics of toileting. He becomes incontinent, loses his balance, the ability to walk, feed himself, to reach for and pick up objects. If he lives long enough without any concurrent illnesses, he will not be able to sit up without support and eventually, not be able to hold his head up. In the late stages of Alzheimer's, the loss of physical abilities can be compared conversely to the acquisition of physical abilities through infancy and childhood. You can frequently look at the behaviors and abilities of a person with Alzheimer's and see a comparison to a child's developmental age. I often used to use these terms when people would ask how Mom was doing, or when my sisters would call to ask what type of gifts to buy for her. I found myself saying, "Well, think in terms of a 5 year old" (or whatever appropriate age). When I teach classes in nursing homes or assisted living facilities, I always tell them you never treat this person as a child, but you do care for him as you would a child. You often get the most favorable results by doing so.

Note, also, that as each ability is lost, it is not actually a physical skill that the person is unable to perform, but rather, the connection between the brain and the legs or hands, for instance, is lost. Often, the skill is lost suddenly, not gradually. When my aunt lost the ability to walk, she could sit with her legs straight out in front of her for half an hour or more at a time. And when you would try to wheel her out of her room and she didn't want to go, she would plant her feet on the doorframe and push herself backwards. She had strength in her legs, but her brain couldn't tell them how to walk any more. When my mother stopped walking (suddenly one day), you could help her up and assist her in walking and she'd go along fine, but she simply could not get up from a chair by herself.

As it turned out, this was a good thing in our case. Mom had been experiencing another relatively uncommon manifestation of Alzheimer's – myoclonal jerking. A few patients experience this. It consists of the whole body involuntarily jerking every little while. Consider what it feels like when you are just barely drifting off to sleep and you dream that you are falling and your whole body jerks. That's what it's like. If the person happens to be standing or walking when it happens, he is liable to fall. In my mother's case, when it began, it would happen every ten minutes or so for about an hour. Finally, it would subside and she'd be exhausted and would sleep. Fortunately, the staff at the nursing home watched the pattern and discovered that it almost always happened in the morning. They would watch her very closely and if it started, they would put her in a geriatric chair till it was over, she'd sleep for an hour or so and then they'd let her go walking again. Unfortunately, over time, it became a more and more frequent occurrence and they had to watch her closely all the time and/or keep her in a geri-chair all the time. As I noted earlier, however, this was about the time that she forgot how to walk. So they were able to put her in a regular chair, she didn't feel like she was trapped, and she was safe because she couldn't figure out how to stand up.

Once the walking slows down, the person can usually focus enough to eat better, but he will probably need assistance. He may eat on his own with just a little help getting started, or he may need consistent coaxing throughout the meal.

If the person has no concurrent illnesses, and Alzheimer's Disease runs its entire course, you will see the person regress through all the stages of childhood, babyhood and infancy. In time, he will need complete care for the activities of daily life. He will need supportive cushioning when in a chair. He will startle easily at sudden movements. (This startle reaction may actually occur much earlier in the disease). The last year or two of his life he will be operating on the level of an infant and will require the same type of care.

People with Alzheimer's do not understand discipline or anger. Studies have been done to show that no matter what physical and mental abilities the person loses, he never loses the emotional component of his personality. He will react emotionally to whatever is going on around him. He will pick up on the mood of his caregivers and respond in kind. And he will become more confused and frightened by negative behavior directed toward him. "It appears that the emotional life of dementia patients is not blunted, but behaviorally and functionally intact to a reasonable degree, even in advanced stages of the disease. Indeed, pre-illness patterns of emotional expression may even become more exaggerated during the course of dementia due to cognitive disinhibition. Symptomatic behavior...may relate to their sensitivity to the avoidance and rejection of others who may erroneously assume that they have diminished capacity to feel. Like pre-verbal infants, they may be even more sensitive to the non-verbal signals of those around them ... because of linguistic impairment, affect remains the only means of communicating wants and needs, likes and dislikes."[5]

On this note, we move to communication skills, keeping in mind that persons with Alzheimer's are always trying to communicate in some manner what they need, what they like, what they don't like. Our task is to interpret that communication.

[1] From an NPR interview with Rudolph Tanzi; co-author with Ann Parson, <u>Decoding Darkness</u>. Perseus Publishing (2000), Cambridge, Massachusetts

[2] Davis, Robert (1989). <u>My Journey Into Alzheimer's Disease</u>, p 92. Tyndale House Publishers, Inc. Wheaton, Illinois.

[3] Excerpts from SPEAKING OUR MINDS: Personal Reflections from Individuals with Alzheimer's by Lisa Anyder, c 1999. Reprinted by permission of Henry Hold and Company, LLC.

[4] Medina, John. (1999). <u>What You Need to Know About Alzheimer's</u>, p.28. CME, Inc.

[5] Magai, C. (2000). Personality and Emotion in Dementia Patients. In <u>Research and Practice in Alzheimer's Disease</u>. Vol. 3, pp 177-181. Springer Publishing Company. New York.

Chapter II

Communication and Care Techniques

"...expressions will change from verbal to nonverbal. We rely on language as the primary vehicle of communication. When behavior begins to speak, it can seem like a whole new language. Begin to listen early in the course of Alzheimer's in the hope that doing so will enhance our understanding. The disease does not result in a complete inability to communicate, but it can require our time, energy and ingenuity to observe, listen and comprehend effectively."[1]

There are two main points that I will keep coming back to in terms of successful interactions with people who have Alzheimer's:

1. Find out who they were before the disease.

2. Go where they are now.

These are the two keys that will make the lives of the caregiver and the one being cared for easier and far less fraught with anxiety and crises. Knowing who this person was in his earlier life will tell you what kinds of things he likes or dislikes, how he has always reacted to situations, what type of work he did, what kind of routine/schedule he is used to, etc. These bits of information can be tremendously helpful in working with him now, as you'll see as we go on.

The second piece of the puzzle is to go where they are now. Once a person reaches a certain stage of Alzheimer's Disease, you cannot bring him into your reality. You have to go where he is because that is the only place you will meet. He will have days and times when he is quite lucid and 'in the moment,' but when he is not, you cannot reason, explain or startle him back to your reality, try though you may. It won't work. I will refer to these two points throughout this and subsequent chapters.

We all have a need to express ourselves, to feel loved and secure, and to be useful. The person with Alzheimer's is no different in this regard, so if you can evaluate the behavior you observe in light of one of these three needs, you'll be better able to respond accordingly. Also keep in mind that if you restrict the person from doing those things of which he is still capable, he will see himself and be seen by others as more impaired than he actually is.

In the earliest days of this disease, talk to the person about his illness and his feelings if he is willing. Personal accounts from people with Alzheimer's suggest that in many cases, the individual would like to talk about his memory problems, but others are not willing to do so. Or others will talk about him in his presence as if he were unable to understand. Talking about the problems at hand can reduce anxiety and help in the acceptance of the situation. However, not everyone is willing nor are they comfortable doing this. That's okay too. Let him set the tone and you follow suit. Perhaps the term 'Alzheimer's' is too disturbing and using words such as 'memory problem' is safer ground. Converse at his pace on whatever level is comfortable.

While the person is still able, it can be beneficial to help him recall his history. Long term memory will be retained for quite a period of time. You should ask him about his past life, and if he seems interested, record it or write it down for him. As a side benefit, you can learn some very interesting things about people. One lady at the nursing home told me about having lost members of her family in a flu epidemic in 1918. She related quite a bit of detail; who contracted it first, and how the children were taken out of the home in hopes they wouldn't catch it, but a couple of them did anyway, herself included. I asked her daughter about this later, and found out that most of what she told me was true. When you didn't have this lady engaged in conversation, she yelled a lot, hallucinated occasionally and often spoke in non-sense terms. But in spite of initial appearances, she still maintained a wealth of information about herself and her past. You can really get a good feeling for people and their lives if you just take the time. Who knows, you may find out things they never told anyone before. "Oral history helps aging patients recover their sense of dignity and purpose. Not only are they encouraged to recover their own past, they also come to take pride in seeing that other people are interested in their lives."[2]

When talking with a person who is beginning to have difficulty expressing himself, it is usually okay to fill in the blanks for him. He is often grateful for the assistance. Also, provide options or negotiate with him to get the best response. If you need the person to do something, rather than giving him the opportunity to say no, offer a couple of suggestions for him to choose from. For instance, "Would you rather wear this sweater or this jacket to go out?" or "Do you want soup or a sandwich for lunch?" This gives him a sense of control. You avoid resistant behavior ("I don't need a jacket." or "I don't want lunch.") and put him at ease when having to answer questions. As the disease progresses, however, you may not want to offer choices any more. It may be too difficult for the person to make decisions. At the point in time when he becomes confused at a two-part sentence or having to make even a simple decision, you should revert to "Here's your jacket." or "Eat your sandwich now."

Talk about the present moment or the distant past. Recalling events in the recent past is difficult, if not impossible, and will cause frustration. If you are helping them to recall the past, don't start your sentences with "Do you remember…" Either get him started by saying "Tell me about your first car." or "When did you first meet your wife?" or else relate an event as if you are telling him for the first time. He will either recall it and join in, or it will seem new to him, and he will enjoy hearing about it from you. Talking about something the person can see or hold is beneficial. Pictures or personal items are good cues for conversation.

Allow the person to perform routine tasks as long as he is able if there is no risk of harm. He needs to feel he has some level of control over his own life, that he is not completely dependent, and that he is useful. So allow him to set the table, clean up after meals, do the dishes, sweep, do minor repairs. At Wesley, one of the tasks they had residents do was to stamp the date on visitors' passes each morning. (It saved the receptionist some work, too). Ask residents to help you clean the lounge or move furniture in preparation for family meetings. Including nursing home residents in daily routines helps them feel ownership of the place in which they live. If they have no tasks to perform, they lose their self-esteem and any sense of purpose.

Paranoia and suspicion are tough issues to deal with. Rarely can you explain things because, as I've noted, 'if…then' reasoning is not accessible any more. Someone says his money has been stolen. You can't say that's impossible because he didn't have any money or because no one has been in his room. That's too logical. First of all, if there was money and you have an idea where his hiding places are, help him look for it. One possibility is that it's a security or control issue you're up against. You could try reaching what is disturbing him. "It must make you very upset to lose your money." or "Has your money been missing before?" or "Let's look for it together." or "We'll find it, but is there something you need to buy right now?" If you stumble on the right question, you may be able to find out where he feels he is losing control and support him in that concern. Or you may be able to 'derail' his train of thought. The main thing is not to deny his suspicions. It will only make him more anxious or angry. Empathize with his feelings. You could alleviate his concern by creating a 'missing items' form that you can help him fill out. In that way, he has a sense of having done something rather than feeling helpless.

In a similar manner, you can meet people's complaints about almost anything head on by agreeing with their anger or annoyance and having them fill out a 'complaint form.' The very creative director of a day care facility said she never allows family members to take the blame for anything. If a participant in the program complains to his family about something at the program or about not wanting to go at all, she instructs them to say, "Go talk to Sue about it." or "Sue said you have to go." If they remember the complaint long enough to talk to her about it, she will have them fill out a complaint form and assures them she will take it to the proper authority. On this same theme, she suggests giving a person who is worried about their money an old bank book. This type of "creative redirection" honors the person and eases a difficult situation.[3]

Anxiety is a common feeling among people with Alzheimer's. Going back to what I said in Chapter I, this is often the result of a person retaining the feeling of an incident long after the actual incident is gone from memory. He can't recall just why, but he knows he is 'supposed' to be worried about something. Occasionally he will remember some details of what occurred, or he may take this distress and apply it to something new or something from his long distant past. The best response, whatever the cause, is to mirror that feeling for him. Tell him you would feel the same if you were in his place. If he can put words to his concern, encourage him to talk about it. Ask questions. "What makes you afraid?" "Have you felt this way before?" If it is a persistent emotion, "Is there any time when you don't feel upset?" Or rephrase whatever they tell you.

One day I encountered a lady walking down the hall of a nursing home, mumbling and grumbling and on the verge of tears. She came up to me and said something unintelligible, but it was clear she was angry and upset. Assuming her tone and expression, I said, "Oh! That's terrible! I'd be upset too if I were you!" She mumbled some more and then clearly said, "Oh! I could have hit her!" And, I said, "Well, I don't blame you! What are we going to do about it?!" She stopped dead in her tracks and looked at me in surprise. She was momentarily derailed because I hadn't patted her on the shoulder and said, "It'll be all right. Everything's fine." She knew I understood her feelings. Of course, I had no idea what was upsetting her, but she didn't know that. I got to where she was and it worked. She quieted down considerably and said, "I don't know what to do." So I said, "How about if you just walk with me a bit and we'll see if we can solve things." We proceeded to walk up and down the hall, and I talked to her about other things, such as the doll she was carrying, and soon she was fine. I told her I had to get going and she said goodbye with a smile.

One sign of anxiety is repetitive hand movements such as rubbing the arm of a chair or patting clothing. This might suggest either restlessness (they need something to do) or over-stimulation (too much noise, light, heat, cold, etc.) Assess the environment and the situation and remove the discomfort to reduce the anxiety.

As this disease progresses, the person will be out of touch with reality more and more of the time. This is the point at which throwing the truth (as we know it) out the window really helps. When my Mother lived with me, I truly believed that as long as I always told her the truth, she would always know that she could trust me, even when she didn't understand. I really tried to live by that premise … and tried … and tried. It doesn't work. And it took me a long time to realize that. Many names have been given to variations of this approach: validation, bent facts, getting into their reality, living their truth, therapeutic lying, illogical logic. But what it all boils down to is going where they are. You are not lying, you are helping. You are trying to walk the path that they are on, and it does work. Oftentimes, it is easier for professional caregivers to do this than it is for family members. There was an elderly lady sitting in the hallway just outside my mother's room. Her daughter was visiting and the woman said, "My mother just died." The daughter replied, "Now, Mother, you know that Grandma died a long time ago." Silence. A few minutes later, "My mother just died." "No, no. Your mother has been dead for years. You know that." This type of exchange went on for quite a while. The lady couldn't give up and her daughter was trying to make her understand. (And let me add here, that at that time in my own caregiving, I would have said the same things. It takes quite a while to learn and put into practice the 'fine art' of letting reality go). Finally, it was time for the daughter to leave. Shortly thereafter, as one of the aides walked by, this lady said, "My mother just died." The aide said, "Oh! I'm so sorry. That must be very sad for you." The woman answered, "Oh, I'm okay, really. But we're going to have to sell her house. I think my brother will take care of things." Then, as an interesting little P.S., the aide said, "How old was your mother?" "81." "And how old are you?" "94." Logic and reason mean nothing. However, the result of this aide's appropriate response was that this lady had her immediate need recognized and she didn't bring it up again.

Don't try correcting the individual. Remember, he is always right and you are always wrong. If you can accept this, battles will be reduced to a minimum. When he asks where his mother/wife/brother is, don't say the person is dead or lives in another state or whatever. Say, 'Gee, I don't know, but where does she usually go this time of day?'[4]

What is one of the most common comments you hear the dementia patient say? 'I want to go home,' or 'take me home.' He will say this whether he is in a nursing home, a day care facility, his son or daughter's home or his own home. 'Home' is a place of security, often the home of his childhood, or just a familiar room. When a person starts asking to go home, there are a few options. Try telling him you will take him but 'how about if we eat first' or do some laundry first or anything that will distract his attention long enough for him to forget. Another option, if circumstances permit, would be to take him out for a walk or for a ride in the car. After a while, he will forget this need to go home and when you return, he will probably recognize this as home. Also, consider solace activities – what can I do to comfort you in this home? Try sorting mail, making a phone call, writing a letter, watching a family video, looking at photos, raking, painting, gardening, yard games like horseshoes, create a birdfeeder or window box. Another idea is to ask him about home. Where is it; what does it look like; who lives there; what did you do when you were there?

Just as an example, there was a relatively new lady in the nursing home whom I encountered in the dining room as dinner was being brought around. She kept calling out to the aides or anyone passing by, "Help me. Can you help me?" So I went over and asked what she needed. She said she needed to go home and could I take her. I said "Sure. Where is your house?" She pointed out the door, "Right there. See it?" I said I did and then asked what color it was. She looked at me as if I had three heads and said "Yellow!" with a tone that said, 'I thought you said you saw it.' So I said, "Oh, yes, okay, I see it now. Why do we have to go there right now?" And then we got down to the point. "My children will be looking for me and if I'm not there, they won't know where to find me." I replied, "Well, actually, they know you're here. They were here yesterday, and they'll come here again looking for you. If you and I go over there, they won't find you." She said, "Are you sure?" and I said, "I'm positive. Now how about we have some dinner and we'll talk about this more later." And she settled right down to dinner. You never know what need or concern is at the source of a comment, but with the right questions, you might just find out. Now there's no guarantee that it won't come up again a while later, but you can always reassure them over again.

One time I sat with a lady who was close to dying. She drifted in and out of sleep and each time she woke, it was with a start and she'd cry out about a fire. Each time I assured her there was no fire, and she'd go back to sleep, but in a fairly restless manner. Finally it dawned on me what I needed to do to reassure this woman. When she woke again and said, "Fire! There's a fire!" I said, "Yes, there was a fire, but the firemen came and put it out and everyone is safe now. See, they're gone and it's all quiet now." She smiled, fell asleep calmly and didn't wake again for quite some time.

It's helpful to know something about the person's background in these types of situations. Supposing you have someone whose work life was in building or construction and he was used to getting up at 4:00 a.m. Now he repeats that pattern, up and dressed at 4:00 a.m. and insisting he has to go to work. Do you tell him he's been retired for years and doesn't have to go to work? No, because he is back in time and he knows better than that. What you do is say that his work crew called and said it's raining at the work site and the job has been called off. Then, "How about if I make you some coffee or you can go back to bed and sleep in." Or for anyone who 'has to go to work,' how about, "The bus is late. Let's read the paper (or whatever) while we wait." Then give him another task to do so as to make him feel like he's working. Here's a creative response. "An art therapist was running a class in which the folks were fabricating things out of tinfoil. She suggested that one of the items looked like an airplane. One participant heard this, looked at his watch, and said, 'I've got to meet Johnson at the airport!' He became insistent that he must leave so they took him to a phone in the office and then fabricated a call to the airport. 'Hello, Johnson, we are wondering what time to meet you at the airport. Oh, not until 8:00 p.m. Okay, we'll be there.' They calmed the man down by explaining they would have to leave in about 4 hours. He was fine and never mentioned it again."[5]

Supposing your family member says, "You never come to see me." Do you say, "Of course I do. I was just here yesterday." No, they won't buy it. How about, "It must be sad to feel like you're alone." That could start a revealing conversation.

If you keep referring back to person's former life, you can really take advantage of his past to help him now. In one nursing home, a new resident gave the staff a really hard time each morning when they tried to get him dressed and going for the day. After a few days of struggling, they talked to his wife and found out that the daily routine at home had been to give him something to eat, a cookie or piece of bread for instance, while she was helping him dress. The staff tried it and was relieved of a lot of stress in this man's care.

What were his lifelong social activities? Again, take advantage of these. Was he a solitary person who enjoyed being alone, or was he gregarious and social? If he was always a solitary person and enjoyed his privacy, don't insist on his joining in on group activities. Give him free rein to spend time in his room with his radio or books or whatever. The natural inclination is to try to get new residents involved and thereby, ward off the depression that often comes with a move to a facility. Check first with family and/or friends. Perhaps this individual isn't depressed, but is content by himself. On the other hand, if you discover that he was a very outgoing, social person, he will not only enjoy group activities, he may enjoy taking part in planning them.

Also, take advantage of his habitual behaviors. The things he has learned to perform by rote throughout his life will be the last to leave. Habits and motor skills which have more or less become part of our core are held onto the longest. I recall one of my aunts who wore dentures. In the morning, if you picked them up, handed them to her and told her to put them in, she couldn't do it. Seeing them out of place and having to follow verbal directions, turned a simple procedure into a complex thought process for her. On the other hand, if you left them on the bedside table, she'd pick them up and put them in automatically because it was a habit.

As stress diminishes (and, by the way, this often happens when a person moves to a care facility where there is a consistent daily routine and there are fewer distractions and changes to deal with) the person will become more compliant to direction. But learn from the past. It may take more effort to get through if he is 'tuned out.'

If an individual is totally focused on some item he is holding or something he is doing and you need him to do something else, try taking his hand or putting your arm around him and gently, but firmly, lead him away. His focus may change as his surroundings change. If you can get him to look at you, try using body language, motion him to follow you. Another possibility is to distract him with a favorite object or toy. Try singing. In any case, as you approach, be sure he sees you before touching him or speaking. If you attempt to stop him abruptly from whatever he is doing, he may become frightened or angry. Ask him what he has. Ask if you could have it, or could he "set it here." If he responds negatively and whatever he has is a danger, take it from him, but replace it with something else. Otherwise, leave him alone for the time being and try again later.

If a person is given to hallucinations, as I stated in the previous chapter, it is harmless unless it frightens him. This is another situation where it is futile to try to give him a lesson in reality. If you want to communicate, you have to go where he is. Two things I have found useful are to go along and say you see the thing or person that he sees, or admit you don't see it and ask what it looks like, what it's doing, etc. Anything that will get these people to talk or express themselves is a means of opening that door to where they are.

Reduce anything in his environment to a minimum when he needs to complete a task such as dressing, bathing or eating. Reduce noise, visual stimuli, other people and provide comfortable lighting and temperature. Too much stimuli leads to confusion and frustration.

If he wants to wear one article of clothing all the time, a particular shirt, sweater or pair of pants, see if you or the family can get a second one just like it so that they can be switched while one is being washed. Accept his clothing preferences. There was a gentleman at the nursing home once who had been a professor and musician, spoke multiple languages, was extremely well educated, loved classical music and fine foods. In his former life he had, more often than not, worn a suit and tie for most occasions. After dementia set in and he moved to assisted care, he was never comfortable unless he had a tie on. He would wear it with pajamas, with t-shirts, with sweatshirts, whatever. The rest of his clothing didn't seem to be an issue, but he didn't feel right without the tie.

When you are assisting someone at mealtime, don't stand over him. It's intimidating. Sit down so you are at eye level. A lady at the nursing home was wheelchair bound and if you sat down and talked to her as you fed her, she was very cooperative. But if the aides were in a bit of a hurry and one of them tried to feeding her while standing, this lady would take the food in her mouth and, when you least expected it, she'd spray it all over. Her favorite thing to do this with was milk. Many a new aide got a milk bath from this little lady.

It may be easier for the person to eat if only one item at a time is put in front of him. A tray full of food, or even a plate full, can be overwhelming. Put a fork or spoon in his hand to see if this will trigger him to eat, or feed him a couple of bites to see if he'll then eat on his own. Offer frequent sips of liquid, particularly if he holds food in his mouth. Give step-wise directions: 'John, here are some eggs. Open your mouth. Chew the food, John. Swallow.' Model what you want him to do. If appropriate, add honey, pudding or sugar to foods not being eaten.

Once the person moves into advanced stages of Alzheimer's, he will require more and more hands-on care. These are the comfort care stages. Particularly for you who are parents, or care for little ones, try to equate the status of each individual with a developmental age. Then offer care – not discipline – accordingly. The standard of care in nursing homes is to treat all patients with dignity and respect as adults; in fact, that which we owe our elders. And this is absolutely valid. You do treat them as adults, however, you care for them as you would a child. There is something to be said for giving the best comfort care that we can.

Here's what a person with Alzheimer's said without sadness or embarrassment; just as a matter of fact. "'I'm becoming more childlike now. I enjoy the things children enjoy. I don't have the same responsibilities. I can do what I want. I really am a child.' His comment was without the disdain I hear from professionals or caregivers who speak of the tragedy of regression to the helpless, incapacitated state of childhood. He recognized an ironic innocence in his simpler life. There were times when his childlike simplicity could be restorative. His wife reports, 'We'll go on a walk and he'll be so excited about a rabbit we might see. On one of our walks, there were a lot of snails on the path and people crushed them as they walked. Bill was stopping and picking up the large ones and throwing them in the shrubs, trying to save their lives.'"[1]

If appropriate care and attention are given, much better responses are elicited and the patient and caregivers are more relaxed. On the other hand, Alzheimer's patients will not respond to typical disciplinary actions such as you would use for a child or baby. These folks are not learning; they're unlearning. Here is a normal, human nature response: "If you don't stop that yelling, I'm going to put you in your room!" or "How many times do I have to tell you not to get into that?" or "If you keep doing that, you're going to fall." Not only does the person have no idea what you're talking about, he doesn't care. Remember there is no logical sequence in his thinking. Trying to point out the consequences of his action has no effect. There is something triggering the behavior. If you can figure out what it is, all the better. If not, just lead him away.

The advantage to caring for an individual as you would a child is in its positive aspects. At four to five years old, a child requires supervision, cannot be left alone, cannot choose clothes or may not dress himself quite properly, and he is very physically active. An Alzheimer's patient with comparable abilities shouldn't be left unsupervised, should be assisted with dressing and bathing, and if possible, should be allowed to walk frequently.

A toddler may act out to test his limits or to express himself over things he has no words for and he may or may not be able to toilet himself all the time. A person with later stage Alzheimer's also acts out by yelling, crying or hitting. His language skills are poor and he may not be able to make his needs known. The major difference here is that it may be easier to discover a two-year-old's needs or intentions. If you know your resident well, you should know what his comfort triggers are – doll, music, dancing, food, pictures, etc. These residents are usually incontinent by this time.

A baby, without proper care, feeding or attention, will cry out. He cannot speak in words nor can he walk. The advanced Alzheimer's patient may cry out for reasons we cannot discern, but there is a need there – and by the way, wanting attention is a legitimate need. They may be hungry, need changing or just rocking. There were two ladies at the nursing home who were fast friends, Mildred and Anna. They spent day after day walking the halls hand in hand. After several years together, Mildred fell and broke her hip and was taken to the hospital and so they were separated. When she came back, she seemed to have lost interest in her old friend. To begin with, she was now in a wheelchair so they couldn't walk together, and she also had family who came to see her regularly. Anna had no one, and she had reached the stage of Alzheimer's where she spoke very little. For a long time afterwards, Anna would periodically give out with this loud, piteous cry that said something was missing and she didn't know exactly what, and she didn't know how to fill that space. The staff and those of us who were there often tried to fill the void; we'd walk with her, hold her hand, talk to her; and she loved that, but it just wasn't the same. And the only way she had to express her sadness was this melancholy cry that came right from her heart.

An infant, without proper hands-on, tender care turns inward to a fetal position and becomes unresponsive. An end stage person will also turn inward, and contract into a semi-fetal position much sooner than he might otherwise. Without the proper care, he will become unresponsive, and stop smiling or making eye contact. You need to provide much physical care, feeding and changing as often as needed. Massage, talking, music and room decorations are helpful as well. In fact, if a person has no concurrent illnesses and does live to this stage of Alzheimer's, a comfort care technique that I thought of and tried at one point is bottle feeding. (I hasten to add here that this option should always be cleared through the care facility's physician or speech pathologist). It occurred to me that as the person goes from regular food to ground food to pureed food, what would be the next logical step? I saw again the reverse comparison to an infant-baby-toddler-child. How is an infant fed before he can be fed with a spoon? With a bottle. When an Alzheimer's patient reaches the stage where he is operating on the level of an infant, it would seem logical that he could take thicker liquids with a bottle. The sucking reflex is retained for some time after other things go. In fact, I once heard at a conference that there is a nursing home – I believe in Virginia, I don't recall exactly – where 'adult feeding bottles' are used for their advanced patients. About a year before my Mother died, she had had a series of difficulties; a bed sore, an infection, flu; and all of this had gotten her down. She wasn't feeling well, she slept a lot, wasn't eating well, but she wasn't in a critical condition. So I thought if I could make it easier for her to take in nutrition during this time, I'd try it. I got a couple of bottles, enlarged the opening in the nipples and gave her thickened juice or high-nutrition drinks (or you could even try milk with baby cereal in it). It worked. When she finally threw off her flu and infections and got her appetite back, she went back to pureed food and juice from a straw, but in the interim, it seemed to be just the thing she needed. Again, whenever there are any issues around swallowing, a speech pathologist is the expert and the first person to contact for evaluation of the patient.

In the final stages of Alzheimer's, you can still communicate. Even though he cannot speak or understand the spoken word, you can still communicate that you care. He is very sensitive to your mood and emotions. Also, keep in mind you can always appeal to the five senses. You can stimulate the person through;

- vision – pictures of familiar things (babies/pets are often a good choice), family photos, colorful things, ceiling decorations for the bedridden
- sound – music, a music box, nature sounds (bird feeder near the window), reading
- scent – flowers, lotion, coffee grounds, wood shavings, cinnamon
- touch – massage, brush hair, do nails, sunshine, soft breeze
- taste – sweets or whatever they like

With regard to room decorations, take note that if the person is bedridden, you need to find things that you can put on the ceiling or high on a window or wall. And notice whether it can be seen from a prone position. Most mobiles or wind chimes are very attractive – if you're standing, looking at them from the side. From below, you don't see much. I put a colorful kite on Mom's ceiling, a rainbow colored sun catcher, and large, magnetic butterflies on the metal strips between her ceiling tiles.

If you play music for him, be sure it is the music of his time and taste, not yours. Modern music doesn't mean anything to him. If you sing or provide tapes of hymns, they should be old, familiar hymns that he would have heard as a boy. Rev. Davis wrote, "…the loudest noise is that which penetrates into my consciousness and rules my perceptions. Modern music … is heard by me only as the beat, accompanied by mingled other sounds."[6]

Scents are an interesting thing. First, you need to make sure that he likes colognes or perfumes and scents and that he isn't allergic to them. (A person who never liked perfumes would definitely not be comforted by them). However, if you can find out if he had a favorite scent (wood chips, coffee, cinnamon?), that would be a plus. Every year, when my father was alive, he would buy my mother gardenias for her birthday, Easter and Mother's Day. The year before my mother died, I recalled this and bought her a gardenia for Mother's Day. These flowers are extremely fragrant and when I brought it in the room and opened the box, its scent filled the room. Mom's eyes got really big and she kept turning toward the source as I moved the flower around. It's hard to know whether it was bringing back a fond memory, but she was smiling all the while. I pinned it to the upper corner of her bed so she'd enjoy it all that day.

General Notes on Communication

In an attempt to help the staff appreciate the residents' backgrounds and interests, one nursing home created collages of what was popular during different decades and hung them on the walls. The residents can easily identify with the pictures and phrases, and the staff becomes familiar with what their elderly patients enjoyed or knew when they were young. When Mrs. Jones doesn't remember being married or having had children, she may be a teenager or a child again. If presented with memories of her era, she will respond very positively.

Let the Alzheimer's person tell whatever is on his mind, and tell it as many times as he needs to. He is looking for some type of confirmation, constantly reassessing his environment to see what is the same and what has changed. Sometimes repetitive statements or repetitive questions, and your responses, are comforting. As frustrating as it may be to give the same answer over and over, you may be helping him keep his feet on the ground.

Help him to think about happier times. If you can find out what circumstances or events made him happy or contented in his former life, you can give that back to him as a gift every single day. I had a hospice patient once who kept trying to tell me about some party or other she had to plan. I discovered that she and her husband had been quite well-to-do and, in fact, entertained often to the extent of putting on lavish galas in hotel ballrooms as well as smaller gatherings in their home. When I figured out the 'game plan,' I would come to visit and ask her to take me shopping. And off we would go – to New York City to shop for dresses in Saks Fifth Avenue or Bloomingdale's. She would ask my opinion on the various colors and designs she was selecting. Or we would plan a whole dinner, along with decorations and invitations. We could enjoy these 'planning sessions' nearly every time I came to visit and she never tired of them.

If you can't understand what he is trying to tell you, watch his body language for clues or look around him to see what he may be referring to.

One day, I was leaving the nursing home after the dinner hour and one of the residents, sitting in a geriatric chair, stopped me. I said "Hi, John. What would you like?" He said, "Well, the guy...and he just ... so I need to ... the thing, cause he took it and never came again." I told him to hold on a minute and went to get a wet paper towel and brought it back to him. He smiled and thanked me graciously. All the while he was speaking, he was making a wiping motion over the tray of his chair. Apparently, one of the aides had taken his dinner away and never cleaned off the tray and it was bugging him.

Be cautious about the words you use. Even though you are dealing with someone who has dementia, he may still be sensitive to the connotation of certain words, because they suggest something childish, or something he finds frightening. For example:

INSTEAD OF	TRY
crafts	project, task
play	exercise, sport
shower/bath	get cleaned up
bib	apron

Also, offer concrete choices when questioning a person. Early on, you can ask multiple choice questions, and later, when the person has difficulty making decisions or sorting out thoughts ask yes/no questions. Open-ended questions will throw the person off and he won't be able to search out an answer. You particularly don't want to ask the type of question that requires he remember the first half in order to answer the second half. You should also give direct instructions, not ask polite questions. For example:

NOT HELPFUL	BETTER
What would you like to wear?	Do you want a sweater or jacket?
Where does it hurt?	Does it hurt here?
Since it's raining, do you want your coat?	Here's your coat
Would you like to come with me?	Come with me now.
Can you sit down?	Sit here.
What would you like to drink?	Would you like water or juice?

Address older people by their proper names early on; Mr. or Mrs. Smith; unless they ask you to use their first names. Use their first names; John or Mary; when they move back in time. This is particularly true of married women. If a woman has regressed to her early years when she was Mary Jones, she won't have any idea who Mrs. Smith is. Use a nickname or title if they respond well; Grandma, Colonel, sir. Be careful here though. I heard 'Grandma' used for various residents at Wesley, and it usually pleased the person. However, one day, an aide referred to a woman as Grandma and she instantly answered, "I have a name you know!"

Don't ask a question he cannot answer. For instance, if you know he was a card player, don't ask if he wants to play cards. Get out a deck and put it down in front of him. He'll respond to the cue.

Always assume he hears you and understands. However, if you make a statement or ask a question and get no response (give him a little extra time to respond) repeat what you said using the exact same words. If you rephrase, using different words, it's basically a whole new concept for him to decipher. If, after two or three repeats, he still doesn't respond, then it's appropriate to rephrase the statement.

Always assume his attempts to communicate are meaningful.

See Appendix A for a series of scenarios in Q & A format addressing how knowledge of a person's background can facilitate his care. Also included are incidents in which you evaluate the cause of a person's behavior; is he trying to communicate, is he insecure, or does he need to feel productive.

---

[1] Excerpts from SPEAKING OUR MINDS: Personal Reflections from Individuals with Alzheimer's by Lisa Anyder, c 1999. Reprinted by permission of Henry Hold and Company, LLC.

[2] Keck, David (1996). Forgetting Whose We Are, p 208. Abingdon Press. Nashville.

[3] Hart, Susan M. (2000). Alzheimer's Society of York Region, Newmarket, Ontario, Canada. Illogical Logic. Talk given at Alzheimer's World Congress, Washington D.C., July 2000.

[4] Brackey, Jolene. (1999). Creating Moments of Joy, p 24. Enhanced Moments. Polk City, IA

[5] Young, Ellen P. (1999). Between Two Worlds, p 112. Prometheus Books. Amherst, New York.

[6] Davis, Robert (1989). My Journey Into Alzheimer's Disease, p 118. Tyndale House Publishers, Inc. Wheaton, Illinois.

Chapter III

Difficult Behaviors

Resistance, confrontation and violence are ways of communicating. The individual who displays these behaviors is looking for something we aren't providing. Unless it is necessary for safety, force should not be used to resolve difficult situations. Trying to determine the cause of the problem can far more effectively calm an aggressive person and possibly prevent this type of occurrence in the future. Also keep in mind that an Alzheimer's patient's ability to understand negative behavior toward himself decreases with time and he can easily become frightened. People with Alzheimer's take their cues from those around them, from their tone and behavior. Interacting in a quiet, calm manner is the best way to handle or avoid difficult behaviors.

Recognize the environmental stressors that may trigger more extreme behavior: unfamiliar place, too many sounds, too loud a sound, bright/flashing lights, no familiar faces, people moving too fast. Try to put yourself in his place. If your senses were limited and you had only a vague awareness of your surroundings, and were unable to think straight, what would help clarify things in your own mind?

"Aggressive elderly persons tend to be more cognitively impaired, more functionally dependent, and have a poor quality of relationships with others. Depressed affect (clinically significant sad appearance) predicted the subsequent onset of physical aggression at some point."[1]

The above quote is from a study which looked at what type of behaviors or occurrences might predict aggressive behavior at a later date. What they discovered was, while certain environmental factors or personality types predicted aggression in some cases, the overwhelmingly common factor in the background of aggressive people was depression. Institutionalization did not affect the outcome one way or the other. Aggression was no more or less likely to start after admission to a care facility than before. However, depression, which is frequently missed in dementia patients, was more often overlooked in people placed in a nursing home. The expectation is that people will have a difficult time adjusting to the nursing home setting and therefore, depressed behavior is 'normal.' It is also looked on as a part of the dementia rather than a separate, treatable condition. The nursing home staff perhaps won't see a difference in the person's attitude and behavior, not having known him before. Those cases which are identified and treated are frequently folks who are at still living at home where family members see a change in behavior above and beyond the dementia. An added complication, however, is that family members may project their own depression on the newly diagnosed individual.

Another predictor of aggression is a person who has always had poor social relationships. This 'personality type' usually is evident long before the onset of dementia. He perhaps never got along well with others, and once confusion sets in, he fights any help or assistance offered. Or he may have had a fairly normal social life, but over time, he pulled away from friends and family and became something of a loner.

Pay attention to signs of deteriorating relationships. Report any signs of clinical depression to a physician. This is a treatable condition that can minimize complications in Alzheimer's.

When you have a person who is prone to violent behavior, try every means to find the cause. Is this a sudden change in behavior for this person? It could be caused by a physical health problem. It is not always easy to recognize acute illness in people with dementia. Persons with visual or hearing loss may perceive emotional events as threatening. Shadows can even cause fear.

Track the pattern of violent behavior; i.e. time of day, during what activity, what triggers these episodes. One fellow in a nursing home was given to violent outbursts about the same time every day. The staff started paying attention to what was occurring just previous to this time and during the time frame in which he was upset. It turned out that a nurse was giving medications at this time and a person from recreation brought a cart to the floor with entertainment and snack items on it. They both parked in the hallway right outside this man's room and residents would come to the two carts for whatever they needed. It was determined that this gentleman was terribly upset that all these people were hovering and making noise in 'his space.' So the nurse and the recreation person moved down the hall to another spot, and the problem was resolved.

Violence could be just a reaction to an accumulation of stress or stimuli, and the person has reached a saturation point. If he is new to a facility, he may be reacting in fear or frustration at not having any orientation cues for finding his room, the bathroom, etc. If this is a long time resident, and the regular staff is at a loss, have someone else look at the situation. A different perspective can help. Limit his choices so he doesn't have to make too many decisions.

Other possible causes:

feeling lost, forgotten

sudden lighting changes

argument between two other people

caregiver's impatience

scolding, contradiction

unexpected physical contact

inability to perform a simple task

activity perceived as too childlike, insulting

Approach an aggressive person with great caution. Do not speak or touch him until he sees you. He may be startled and strike out instinctively. One person should stay with the individual while others move people and objects out of harm's way. If he trusts you, lead him away by the hand or motion for him to follow you if he doesn't want to be touched. Try soothing distraction techniques to relocate the person to a calmer or more familiar environment.

If you can pinpoint an ongoing cause, change the environment and/or his care pattern and make sure all staff is made aware of the change (including temporary caregivers). If cause cannot be determined, experiment with diversions – chewing gum, music, food, solitude, personal photos – or exercise, dancing. If he won't let you near him, keep a safe distance away and talk to him about objects in his room; photos, wall hangings, the clothes he is wearing. Just try to get him to focus on something else momentarily. I heard of a situation once where a man would have aggressive episodes and if one aide stood in front of him to hold his attention, another would come behind him and gently place ear phones on his head with classical music playing. He would calm right down.

He may not like a particular aide or gender. One time a gentleman had come to the nursing home and a male aide was assigned to him. Each time he would go into the man's room, the man would become angry or would cower as if he were afraid. Finally, one day, when the aide came in, he said something to the effect of, "You go away! You're not going to hurt me!" After doing some investigation, it was discovered that this man had been a prisoner of war during World War II and for some obscure reason, he saw this particular aide as a German prison guard. Clearly, he had gone back in time to those terrible days during the war. What he saw in this particular aide that prompted the fear is anybody's guess. He was reassigned a female aide and did very well with her.

Occasionally a firm "What do you want?" or "I know you are angry!" is enough to get his attention and break the cycle. "If you witness a gentleman who is upset or two men fighting, walk up to them and extend your hand for a handshake and ask if there is anything you can do to help. A handshake is a friendly gesture that brings down a wall and men respond very well to it."[2]

Reduce aggression by improving the person's sense of safety, physical comfort and control. Minimize stress and maximize pleasure. If you know this person well, you should have an idea what his stressors are. If you don't, you'll have to be creative. Accept his reality. Keep trying to put yourself in his place. Also keep in mind that what works one time may not work another, or what works for one person may not work for another. After the episode is over, reassure the person that you understand and care. It was probably as frightening and upsetting to him as it was to you.

If you have to perform a physical exam or do some type of physical care for a person who fights and is resistant, try these steps. Enter his room as if you are a friend or visitor. Sit down to achieve eye level. Chat with him for a couple minutes – admire clothes, jewelry, pictures, etc. Typically, a person with dementia will be very trusting and this gives him a chance to feel like he knows you. Next, introduce the steps of the exam one at a time. "How about if I check your heart now?" Show him the stethoscope. If possible, remain seated. "Now I'm going to take your pulse." Continue in this way so that your movements and directions don't become overwhelming. Even from a 'normal' perspective, consider any time you have had dental work or minor surgery. You are in a reclined or prone position with people standing over you with heaven knows what kind of instruments. It's intimidating. All the more so if you couldn't understand what was being done to you.

Violent behavior can be the result of a downward cycle of events. If this is recognized early on, it can be stopped. Rev. Davis describes it this way, "I cannot stand the beat of rock music or the bouncing around of senior citizen aerobic classes. Human dignity demands that I have the right of refusal for any activity or entertainment that I do not perceive as entertaining. I could never bear to be talked to and treated like a child at summer camp. I am repulsed by some 20 year old trying to get me to play childish exercises to rock music. I'm sure I would try to get back to my room and if stopped in this attempt I would become belligerent. If she continued to push or became condescending and began to pat my arm, I would probably explode. If I were then restrained or tied in my chair, my fury would take me right out of my mind."[3]   This is a good description of how a person could get caught up in a cycle of violence that he couldn't easily get out of unless others see the pattern and break it.

Yelling

This is often seen in advanced Alzheimer's patients, those who are physically immobile and have lost the ability to speak. They are trying to communicate their needs, thoughts, etc. Sometimes this is a habit the person no longer has control over. They may just like the sound they are repeating over and over because it is rhythmic.

Other possible causes:
> hunger, need for bathroom
> uncomfortable position
> inability to be understood
> too much/not enough stimulation
> restraints
> upset by other residents

Check for all possible physical solutions first. Then create a relaxed atmosphere. Reduce noise, lower lighting, read to him, play soft music. Maintain a very consistent routine for these folks. Try having a staff member go in to the person's room every half hour or so and spend five or ten minutes talking to him whether he is yelling or not. If it's a difficult patient whom no one likes to care for, all staff can take turns spending time with him. The patient may become habituated to these visits, recognize that he will get attention whether he yells or not, anxiety will decrease and yelling may decrease.

Try giving him a project depending on his ability – mending, folding sorting, putting paper clips in a box or jar, fixing something (have simple toys or such on hand that can be taken apart and reassembled fairly easily), sorting or playing cards. Get the family to make a tape of their voices speaking, reading or singing and play it when the resident is anxious.

Wandering

Wandering is a restlessness caused by changes in the brain, anxious feelings, the physical comfort of movement, or a search for something familiar. Often it is caused by previous work roles, or it may be a method of coping with stress. Find out what type of work the person did, what his personality was like and what his response was to stress when younger.

Other possible causes:

> too quiet, boredom
> looking for light
> feels closed in, trapped
> familiar person is out of sight
> confusion between dreams and wakefulness
> anticipation of an event

Obviously, if the environment allows it, let him walk. It's actually good for the individual with Alzheimer's. He works off excess energy and anxiety and may sleep better. It's been found that he will remain a little more aware and physically capable for a longer time when he exercises. Rev. Davis: "I would ride on an exercise bicycle until I was exhausted and my mind was clear. ...physically demanding activity. Following this, I rest quietly and sometimes fall asleep. When I wake, I am refreshed and usually more alert mentally."[4]

In terms of prevention, don't tell the person when an event is coming up until you are practically on your way out the door. If you plant the thought that they have an appointment or luncheon or some other occasion to attend, the details will be lost, but the sense of having to go somewhere will become pressing. He will pace, he will question, he will try to go out. Even though we often say anticipation is half the fun, anticipation is not an enjoyable thing for a person with Alzheimer's. Keep items out of sight that trigger a desire to go out; boots, coat, purse, etc.

Involve him in housekeeping activities. In an assisted living facility, make sure the family provides familiar objects for his surroundings. Perhaps they could bring a large digital clock. If he wakes during the night, seeing the time may help orient him. Try written reassurance. Give him a note to carry saying, "Mary will be here at 2:00." Try showing him photo albums or travel books.

Once the wandering has begun, try to find out where they are going. When my Mother would take off in the middle of the night, my husband would follow her down the street and ask where she was going. She'd say to Church or the store and he'd say, "Okay, but come on back and I'll drive you." Often, by they time they walked back to the house, she'd have forgotten her mission and come right in. If this didn't work, you could put the person in the car and drive him around the block and it may be enough to satisfy him. If not, drive by a closed store and say, "Well, it looks as if it's closed. We'll come back tomorrow."

If he is trying to 'escape' from a facility, ask him where he is going and why. Get him to talk to you, if possible. You may find out what is prompting his need to wander and be able to feed that need, or you may just get him sidetracked and talking about something else. Whenever possible, guide the conversation around to what is pleasant to him. For instance,

"Where are you going?"

"I have to go to work."

"Oh really? What time do you have to be there?"

"8:00." (You could tell him it's not time yet ...)

"What do you do at work?"

"I'm a foreman."

"Wow. That's a pretty responsible position. How many people work for you?"

"Ten."

"Are they all pretty good workers? How do you manage them?"

Can you see this conversation turning itself around to a discussion of what he did as a younger man when he felt useful and needed? That may be all it takes to turn a person from his course and fill the need he has at that moment: remind him of how important he was – and still is.

A person who wanders within the building just because he needs to keep moving can be managed a bit easier. Again, let him walk the halls. At meal time, don't try to seat him until dinner is actually there. If you keep trying to get him to sit in preparation for dinner, he will just keep getting up and/or become so frustrated that when the food comes, he won't be able to focus and eat. Another option, if it is workable, is to give him food to carry as he walks. When he reaches the point where he doesn't know it's food in his hand and starts leaving it around various places, try to give him bites of food each time he comes through the dining room. You're not teaching him bad habits. He isn't learning; he is unlearning. 'This too shall pass.'

Rev. Davis: "When darkness and emptiness fill my mind, it is totally terrifying. I cannot think my way out of it. The only way I can break this cycle is to move."[5]

Alzheimer's patients must live within boundaries of comfort and control. Those boundaries get smaller as time goes on. Maintain a quiet, calm atmosphere, reducing stimuli wherever possible. As I stated earlier, all of the caregiving and interaction skills given here come back to one of two things; who was this person before Alzheimer's and where is he now? If you can tap into his history and walk with him now, you will give him moments of joy and a real sense of security and being understood.

[1] McShane, R., Cohen-Mansfield, J., Werner, P. (2000). Predictors of Aggressive Behaviors. In Research and Practice in Alzheimer's Disease, Vol. 3, pp. 183-188.

[2] Brackey, Jolene. (1999). Creating Moments of Joy, p 142. Enhanced Moments. Polk City, IA.

[3] Davis, Robert (1989). My Journey Into Alzheimer's Disease, p 102. Tyndale House Publishers, Inc. Wheaton, Illinois.

[4] ibid, p 96

[5] ibid, p 96.

Chapter IV

Caring for the Family

<u>For Nursing Home/Care Facilities</u>

Families can be the greatest asset or the greatest liability to a nursing home staff. Typical family impressions or expectations upon placement of their loved one are "These people don't know my loved one and can never take care of him as well as I do." or "These people are professionals and I know my loved one will get excellent one-on-one care 24 hours a day." The typical, but perhaps subconscious, attitude of the staff is, "We're professionals. We've been doing this for years. We'll get this new resident settled in, blend him into the group and hope the family is agreeable."

With these kinds of viewpoints, this relationship may be headed for conflict, and misinterpreted actions. "Each time you admit a resident to your facility, you are admitting that resident's family as well. Those family members can be your most ardent supporters or your most cutting critics. Resident care with a family centered focus will go a long way to establishing your facility as one that values the importance of maintaining family integrity, even in the face of nursing home placement."[1]

The family may feel it is relinquishing its duties and breaking a sacred promise by placing a loved one in a nursing facility. They are no longer living up to what they believed to be their responsibility. This guilt may be manifested by being overprotective or unjustifiably critical. They may refuse to visit or else be there constantly, complaining about every aspect of care.[2] The family may not know what to do with themselves when the caregiving burden is lifted.

They are stressed, tense, guilty, relieved, overly expectant. Deal with them gently. They have been stretched emotionally, physically, financially and socially. There's not much left that's not vulnerable.

Starting with the admission process, all the steps in nursing home placement can lead to a smooth transition for everyone involved. The day a family brings their loved one into the facility, be there for them. Have several staff members meet the family and greet the new resident. Answer questions and offer information on the day to day life in the facility. Guide the family and resident through the process and reassure them that you will answer their questions again and again as they try to absorb all the new information.

Do not leave the new resident alone on the first day! He will need a great deal of reassurance, particularly after the family has left. Provide for a social worker, aide or someone to be sure that he is comfortably occupied all throughout this day. Introduce him to one or two other residents who have rooms nearby or who are compatible in terms of the level of dementia each one has. Call the family later in the day or encourage them to call you so that they will be reassured that their loved one wasn't forgotten as soon as the family left.

In the first few days after admission, give a little extra attention to the new resident. Assist at his meals initially. The activities of the floor may be routine to you, but they can be traumatic for the resident and/or family. One resident who came to the floor my mother was on, came from another part of the facility where there was less hands-on care and supervision. It was assumed that since she had been on the campus for a time already, she didn't need any type of orientation. Therefore, the staff treated her like a long-time resident. Unfortunately, the family felt their mother was being ignored. Because it was, in fact, a new environment for the woman, her confusion increased, she had some difficulty settling in and she stopped feeding herself. She would eat well if someone sat with her for a bit and encouraged her to start, however, no one but her family did this for her. What may seem like old hat to you can be very stressful for the resident and family. When my mother arrived at Wesley, they were overwhelmingly kind to us. My mother was restless back then and wanted to walk all the time and get outside often. During those first couple weeks, anyone who happened to be available when she was overcome by this need to get out would go with her, walk her around the block and bring her back. This turned out to be just enough and she would come back in willingly. Many people walked her – an aide, social worker, chaplain, nurse – everyone was extremely nice in accommodating new residents. She settled down within the first couple weeks and the daily 'needed' walks disappeared. I was greatly comforted that no one was fighting her on this issue.

The family or primary caregiver of a new resident may have lost touch with normal life and may not realize his or her needs. Encourage the family to talk about how they are feeling. If you have one available, show a film or share a booklet on what to expect when it comes time for nursing home placement. There will be guilt, anger and all sorts of disrupted emotions on the part of both the resident and his family. They need to know that this is normal.

Have the various services contact the family to inquire as to the resident's interests or needs or send an 'interest information sheet' home to the family to fill out. Then act on the information you have acquired to the best of your ability.

Throughout the resident's stay, the staff on the floor can provide positive feedback to the family. This can come from the social worker and administrative personnel as well. The folks who will interact with the family most of the time can give them a sense of confidence that they have made the right decision and that their loved one is safe and sound. I had placed my mother in another facility before moving her to Wesley, and during that short time (two weeks), every time I went to see her, morning, noon or night, the staff would complain about her. "Your mother got out of the building!" (Who wasn't watching her?) "If she doesn't stop doing that, we're going to have to tie her down." (You do and the state will be in here faster than you can blink). "Your mother keeps putting her things on her roommate's bed!" "She keeps taking the sugar packets off the tray and hiding them." You would have thought this staff had never seen someone with Alzheimer's before. And this was a dementia-specific unit! (My impression was that their way of coping was the use of serious tranquilizers, although I could be wrong). I called my sister one day and said, "I have this sinking feeling that one of these days I'm going to get a call asking me to take her out of there." There was one nurse on nights who was nice to us. After about four or five days, she told me that she thought Mom was adjusting quite well considering the short time she had been there. With the exception of that one woman, whom, unfortunately, I didn't see too often, it was a most miserable and stressful experience.

Host family get-togethers or holiday gatherings, by floor or by unit. Not only is this a good social occasion between families and staff, but it helps families to become acquainted with each other.

Provide educational talks or programs on financial, legal or health issues for instance.

Put new families in touch with other experienced, supportive family members.

Always provide avenues of recourse to the family – phone numbers, updated staff lists.

Offer a family council group where information and issues can be exchanged and discussed.

Ask the family about all aspects of the resident's life before admission and, more importantly, before the disease. This will improve their sense of contribution and your caregiving skills. While certain caregiving skills are uniform across the board, each individual resident will respond in his own way to certain things; certain foods, routines, activities. Help to optimize his enjoyment of his new home. Also, the family appreciates the opportunity to talk about the past. Relating who this person was before Alzheimer's is a welcome reminiscence for them.

One facility in Iowa City, Iowa has what they call a "Partnership Agreement."[2] This is a document that is drawn up for each new resident and renegotiated periodically. Some of the items asked of the family for inclusion in this document are;

- What would be helpful for the staff to know?
- How would you like to be involved in care?
- Can we provide instruction/training?
- What are the resident's needs; how can they be met?
- How can the staff support family involvement?

Ask the family to make audio or video tapes for their loved one to hear when they are not present. This is especially helpful for residents who speak or have reverted to a foreign language. Also ask them to bring photos or scrapbooks.

Encourage family involvement and visits. Let them know when the resident needs clothes, shampoo, etc. Provide 'visiting kits' for uncomfortable family members to borrow. These are little collections of items such as old familiar ads, or items associated with sewing or carpentry or the four seasons, or photos of older clothing styles. Cards or photo albums may help initiate conversations or activities with residents who have dementia.

Ask the family member's opinion on optional care issues, such as going to an on-sight hairdresser/barber, or the best time to settle him down for the night. Train the family in skills and knowledge of resident care. If the family hasn't had any experience in hands-on care, or the staff isn't comfortable with having their help, shift the focus to resident success. If everyone has this as the goal, working together will go more smoothly.

Remember to take the family step by step through the caregiving process at a pace they are comfortable with. They may only be comfortable assisting at mealtime, or they may want to assist with all caregiving activities. Often family caregivers are not accepted as part of the health care team, but can be expected to do things they are unprepared for. When they are comfortable with a team approach and confident in their ability to relate with persons with dementia, family members may even interact and assist with other dementia residents. The family can enhance the staff's ability to provide individualized care of the resident, and the staff can enhance the family's ability to assist in physical care.[3]

View the family as assisting to relieve staff overload, as a source of useful information about the resident, and as people who need sensitive attention right along with the resident, especially in the early days of placement. Family members feel sad over the relative's deterioration, powerless in an institutional setting, guilty and perhaps they are having difficulty readjusting their home lives without the loved one.

Inform the family of all medical concerns and changes. More often than not, one of the family members has power of attorney and is the health care proxy and should be allowed to have input in all medical/medication decisions, or at the very least, be informed of what decisions are being made with regard to her loved one. Besides her right to know, she is probably the person most involved in day to day observation of the individual and can report any changes that occur before or as a result of medical/medication changes.

As the person with Alzheimer's becomes incontinent, loses his ability to speak, to walk, to feed himself, etc., he becomes far easier to care for. He cannot complain; he cannot ask for things; he doesn't need to be taken to the bathroom; he cannot get into things. In effect, he also becomes far easier to ignore. Family members are keenly aware of this. They become the only voice the resident has at this point, and if it seems they are becoming more and more insistent about care issues, it is because they sit by the bedside and see staff members responding to the residents who are yelling, who are into others' rooms, who want attention, who need to go to the bathroom. It is so easy to walk by the room of the person who makes no noise and can't get out of his bed or chair. It's easy to let him sit or lie in one position for long periods of time. Why take the time to get him a blanket or sweater? After all, he didn't say he was cold. These are the folks who, ideally, should want for nothing. When all that is needed for superior care is to be warm, clean, dry and fed, there is no excuse for ignoring these things. Give these residents extra TLC and then tell the family, each time they come in, what you have noticed lately about their loved one, what seems to content him, what you avoid because it disturbs him. This extra awareness of his humanity and sharing with the family will go farther in building good will than anything else you can do.

End of Life Issues

(Also see Chapter V on Hospice Care)

The family will need more attention in the end stages of this disease. When their loved one is dying, they need to know that he is being watched closely and that they are being supported in their vigil. Too often, I've heard families say they sat by the bedside hour after hour and no one came by. Naturally, they see this as lack of caring on the part of the staff, when, in fact, the staff may feel they shouldn't disturb the family. They avoid going in the room mistakenly thinking;

- they don't want to get in the way
- hospice has come in and they aren't needed
- there is nothing to be done for the patient

If the resident has been living in this facility any length of time, the regular staff has become like family to him. They should be allowed to grieve this upcoming loss also. Not only does the family need extra support at this time, but they will be touched to think that you share in their grief. Even though hospice may have been brought in, the regular staff members are the ones who know this person and this family. Your familiar presence is needed too. Talk to the family about the resident and what he meant to you.

Ask about his former life before he came to the facility. Families almost always appreciate an opportunity to talk about their loved one.

Typically, the family feels immense support by just having people stop in briefly, but frequently. Ask if there is anything they need. And if they ask that something in particular be done for the resident, if it's not harmful, <u>do it</u>. At this point, you are caring for the family as much as you are the patient, and if some simple service will give that family member some ease in their distress, you do it. One daughter of a resident at the nursing home sat by her mother's bedside, watching this woman thrash about, restlessly moving until she was way over by the side of the bed. The daughter rang for assistance and when the staff member came in, she asked for help in moving her mother back to the center of the bed where she'd look more comfortable. The staff member said no; there was no point; it wouldn't help her; she'd only move back to the side again anyway. You can imagine how stressful this would be for a family member.

On the other hand, I sat with a family whose father was comatose. At one point, someone called for a nurse and said she thought he looked uncomfortable but she didn't know what to do. The nurse gently swabbed his mouth and took a cool washcloth and wiped his face and hands. Subsequently, this nurse came in about every half hour and repeated this procedure. To this day, that family has nothing but gratitude for this woman who genuinely cared for their father and empathized with their grief. We don't know if it made a difference to the man who was dying, but what a gift to that family!

Family Members of Those Without Dementia

What about the families of those residents who do not have Alzheimer's? How can you help them? These folks encounter the dementia patients every time they visit. They probably won't be comfortable around them, nor know how to deal with them. In addition, they will be even more distressed if they perceive their family member as being 'victimized' by the Alzheimer's residents.

It can take some time before a person becomes comfortable around dementia patients, but the more information they have, the more likely they are to make this transition. Totally aside from dementia patients, most people can't 'get past the wrinkles' or the nursing home environment at all. How often I've heard people comment, "It's so sad to see those poor 'things' just sitting there." Now they have a family member residing there and are committed to coming to visit.

Encourage them to spend time, to come at mealtime and help out, to take their family member into the dining or living room. It's the only thing that is going to help them see that this is not a terrible place, but a very interactive community of people. In time, they will see that generally, the residents within a wing or floor become a family, all the various personalities interacting – worrying about one another, fighting, laughing, living together. And those "poor things just sitting there" are probably sitting near the nurses' station or the elevators watching the world go by. These are the two spots where all the action is. Okay, so sometimes they doze off and fall asleep on the job. That's okay too. The elderly, demented or not, don't need to be running around looking for all sorts of activity and entertainment all the time. Their environment has naturally decreased with age and would have whether they were at home or here. There is a comfort in the security and routine of a nursing home if it is a good one where the staff truly cares.

Encourage families to come often, to get as involved as they are comfortable with and to get a sense of this place as home. Frequent exposure plus some education can move most people past that invisible line of resistance. They will be able to look from the inside out rather than the outside in.

Provide family members with training on communication and interaction skills with dementia patients. This could be in the form of one-to-one suggestions from the floor staff or in a family council setting where someone could come in to do a presentation for them. If family members can learn some simple basics, they will be much more comfortable visiting. Some of the topics which should be covered are;

- a general overview of what dementia is
- how to 'go where they are' or get a sense of the resident's reality
- how to get their attention and speak to them
- some techniques for distracting or redirecting the resident
- how to transfer their attention to a staff member

It's possible with some of the more frequent and active visitors that you may get a bit of assistance from them if they don't mind having the dementia residents around.

Try to be proactive about keeping dementia residents out of other residents' rooms. This can be a difficult task, but very significant in maintaining good will. Sometimes it only requires a closed door, or an eye-level net or something with fringe to get them to turn around. You know who your wanderers are – try to keep them in community areas or keep them busy with folding/sorting tasks when you can't watch them. Whenever any staff member goes down the hall, glance in the rooms as you go by to check for 'unwanted visitors.' Consider how unfair it is to those who are mentally alert but physically limited. They are being penalized in the sense that they cannot keep nice things around their rooms for fear they will be taken or broken.

An aggressive resident can harm the more frail residents. He may have no intention to harm, but he doesn't realize his own strength or, perhaps is trying to help someone to stand or move about when the individual cannot do so. These folks must be watched and controlled at all times. If there is no one free to accompany this resident, bring him where you are. Provide him with activities and plenty of exercise as appropriate so as to use up energy and encourage relaxation.

Also see Chapter VII and Chapter VIII for more information on family and caregiver issues.

---

[1]Geffen Mintz, Suzanne. National Family Caregivers Association. Quoted in The Council Close-Up: Illinois Council on Long Term Care. No. 161, 5/24/1996.

[2] Springer Brenneman, Dianne; Pringle Specht, Janet (1996). Family Involvement in Care Study, University of Iowa, Iowa City. Family Involvement in Care: Family/Staff partnerships in Special Care Units. Presentation, 5th National Alzheimer's Disease Education Conference. Chicago, Illinois.

[3] Belle, Cynthia. Kavanaugh, Kevin. Blake-Curry, Kathleen. (2000). Proactive Management of Family Adjustment to Long-Term Care. Presentation given at World Alzheimer's Congress. Washington, D.C. July 2000.

Chapter V

Hospice Care*

Until fairly recently, hospice was not an option for patients with Alzheimer's Disease. One of the requirements for admission to a hospice program is a prognosis of six months or less. However, depending on concurrent conditions, this disease can last from 2 to 20 years or even more. Making a terminal diagnosis is difficult. The patient is usually unable to report his symptoms and may have a decreased sensitivity to pain. Also, medical decisions must be made without input from the patient.

In addition to those barriers, the orientation of hospice has always been a family-based mode of care which includes enhancing the patient's life. Because of the nature of Alzheimer's Disease, the patient may seem to the hospice team to be almost inaccessible. By the time hospice enters the picture, there may be no conversation with the patient, no opportunity to fulfill any of his needs or wishes. There may be little or no social or personal interaction. Generally, pain management is not needed. With regard to the family, typically the hospice team assists them in dealing with the shock and anticipatory grief of a terminal diagnosis. The Alzheimer's family has probably been dealing with this illness, and all the issues surrounding it, for years. Grieving may have been worked through or set aside. Also, because of the length of this disease, the nursing home staff or family may be resistant to hospice 'taking over.'

However, in the recent past, the thinking on this has changed. Taking into consideration concurrent conditions or illnesses, patients can be evaluated so as to determine a six month prognosis. First, the physician looks at the stage of Alzheimer's the person has reached in terms of the patient's ability to perform activities of daily living; dressing, feeding, toileting, etc.; his speech patterns, mobility and continence. The individual is rated according to various scales such as independent to completely dependent or regular to disrupted. Along with these ratings, he will also look for concurrent problems such as susceptibility to infectious illnesses or pneumonia, recurrence of urinary tract infections, decubitus ulcers (bedsores), unexpected weight loss, difficulty swallowing or eating. Of course, if there is a serious concurrent illness as well, such as cancer or heart disease, this will be the primary determinant of the person's eligibility for hospice.

The decision to move a loved one into a hospice program must be made by the family, but again, at this stage of the illness, the family has been making all medical decisions in the absence of the patient's ability to do so. They will need to be counseled as to exactly what hospice will offer and do for their loved one. If they believe this is the right step, they must also be reassured that they can change their minds at any time and take him off the program. Perhaps two of the major points on which this decision turns are whether or not to give antibiotics for infections and whether or not to provide assisted nutrition and hydration. These were key in my decision making. As to the first, I felt that if my mother were to get pneumonia or some type of infection, by withholding antibiotics, we would be introducing a new cause of death. She was already dying of Alzheimer's, and that I accepted. I didn't accept the idea of hurrying that process along by allowing an easily treatable condition to go unchecked. More than a year before my mother died, she had a bedsore at the base of her spine. One doctor (who, fortunately, was not her doctor) suggested we not treat the bedsore, let it have its way and let 'nature take its course.' Thankfully, neither her caregivers, nor myself, saw it that way. They treated the problem aggressively and returned her skin to a healthy condition in a remarkably short time. By the same token, if she had had several bouts of pneumonia or skin ulcers and had come to the point where the antibiotics did not help, then fine. In that case, treatment would be without purpose.

With regard to assisted nutrition and hydration, (they are usually called "artificial" nutrition and hydration), families are often told that this is not a good idea, that IV fluids or tube feeding will only prolong the dying process and will probably make him more uncomfortable. While this is true in some cases, it seems to me that it is far too prevalent an attitude and is pressed upon families across the board rather than on a case by case basis. I volunteered with a hospice patient who had a stroke while in the nursing home. He no longer spoke or moved or ate. The hospice and nursing home staff told his wife that it was best that she let him go. He wouldn't want to live like this. She told me that she just wasn't comfortable with this decision. It didn't feel right. She couldn't bear to watch him become more and more dehydrated. I told her she was free to take him off hospice any time she wanted and since she was his wife, she should do whatever felt right to her. This man was in her heart and the staff couldn't make decisions about that. Two days later, when I came in to see him, I discovered she had requested he be transferred to the hospital for hydration. I went over there and found her sitting contentedly beside his bed. He was still unresponsive, but not struggling to breathe as he had been. She said that even if he died now, she was satisfied that she had done the right thing. He just looked so much better to her. Three days later, he was awake and responsive and she took him home. I called her a couple days later and she said he was so happy to be home, she realized that he had 'given up' after his stroke because he was depressed over being in the nursing home. I wasn't in touch with them after that, because he was off the hospice program, but about a year and a half later, I saw his death notice in the paper; a year and a half that this couple had together in their own home because she chose not to 'let nature take its course.'

I debated at length about what I would do when my mother reached the point of not being able to take nutrition on her own and finally, a good friend offered this. If not eating will be the cause of death, assisted nutrition and hydration are called for. If not eating is part of the dying process, let it be. I think that's a pretty fair balance when it comes to making this type of decision for someone who is mentally incapacitated. As it turned out, Mom started noticeably losing weight before she stopped eating. This was a clear sign that her digestive system was shutting down, so there was no question in my mind that assisted nutrition was not appropriate.

Hospice staff should be able to help the family to make an informed decision about these issues. So, going back to my original premise, a six-month prognosis can now be made for patients with dementia. Subsequently, decisions need to be made by the family and the hospice team, (and a nursing home staff if applicable). The family makes the team aware of the needs and wants of the patient if they were expressed before dementia, as well as their own ethical requirements. The hospice team contributes the best in palliative care on a case by case basis. Hospice and the nursing home should then work together to create a new care plan for the resident emphasizing comfort care rather than rehabilitation or restorative care. What then, does hospice have to offer the Alzheimer's family?

- The patient's own doctor can remain in charge.

- A licensed hospice nurse to oversee the care of the individual

- A certain number of hours of personal aide service

- A social worker will be available for the family.

- Pastoral care and counseling

- Medicare coverage as well as coverage of medical equipment and medications

- Volunteers to visit, run errands, offer moral support, sit with the patient, etc.

Ideally, before any of this takes place, the hospice staff should undergo dementia-specific training. All members of the team, from the volunteers to the doctors, are most likely used to dealing with cancer cases, occasionally AIDS, perhaps heart or renal failure. However, both the dementia patient and the family will, in many ways, have very different needs than any of these. The following, in conjunction with the previous chapters of this book, can provide hospice staff with the tools they need to assist Alzheimer's families.

The Disease Process

Alzheimer's Disease begins to manifest itself through random, occasional memory lapses which are not typical of the individual. These memory lapses become more and more frequent until concern drives the person or their family to seek a diagnosis. For a fairly long period of time, the individual will be quite aware of what is happening because a good part of the time, he is lucid and capable. Eventually, the occasional memory lapses will become all encompassing and the lucid moments will become random and occasional. In time, he moves into that 'other world' wherein he no longer is conscious that there is a problem.

Over a span of two to twenty years or more, besides losing intellectual functions, he will also gradually lose the ability to carry out routine activities and his physical mobility will be lost. Each physical loss, however, is not initially an actual physical incapacity, but rather a gap in the messages that the brain sends to the various parts of the body. For instance, a person who cannot walk probably lost that ability suddenly, and can, in fact, walk with assistance. On his own, however, he has forgotten how. The brain can no longer send a message to the arms, torso and legs to stand up, and put one foot in front of the other.

At the point in time when hospice enters the patient's life, he may be immobile, unable to speak and may also be bedridden. On first observation, one would assume that death is imminent. Surprisingly, however, this stage of Alzheimer's can last for two or three years. The Alzheimer's patient regresses through the stages equivalent to childhood, babyhood and infancy. Eventually, as the brain shuts down various bodily systems, the body is no longer able to function and the lungs and heart will give out. Fortunately, in most of the cases that reach this stage of the disease, little or no pain is experienced. The person just appears to weaken with each day and dies rather peacefully.

The Caregiving Experience

By the time the Alzheimer's family opts for hospice, the caregivers have experienced an entire range of reactions:

- physical – occasional assistance has become full time care
- emotional – shock of diagnosis, anticipatory grief, anger, guilt, fear
- financial – especially for spousal situations
- social – isolation, misunderstanding (early on, patient looks normal), people don't come ('He won't know me anyway')

The grief this family has experienced has gone through all the stages, perhaps many times over: shock, denial, anger, depression, sleeplessness, guilt, anticipated loss, acceptance. This is compounded by the ongoing situation and losses. The family is misunderstood, their difficulties minimized, and there may be little tolerance or sustenance for their grief. The community cannot sustain someone's grief over such a long period. Neither can the individual. Placement in a nursing home can represent "permanent severing of attachment bonds. There are no rituals, no public acknowledgement, no expressions of sympathy to support feelings of loss."[1] This is particularly keenly felt by spouses. As a result, one needs to 'normalize' the situation. The family will, of necessity, have reached some level of acceptance; this life has become the 'norm.' When hospice comes into the picture, there will be some fear of the loss of routine or what has become normal for this family.

In spite of the length of time this illness has gone on, or perhaps because of it, the introduction of hospice may give the caregiver a sense of disbelief and shock. The first couple years of coping with Alzheimer's entail a lot of anger and guilt and denial. In time, the caregiver recognizes that this is an unbeatable disease and their loved one will die, probably soon; certainly within another year or two. But he doesn't and thinking is readjusted again. When the situation becomes normalized, she eventually assumes that it will always be this way. It will never change. The patient may change in terms of his physical and mental status, but he will always be there in one condition or another. There is typically a calm acceptance at this point and the relationship between the caregiver and patient moves to a new and different level. The caregiver puts the past totally away and lives in the present reality, caring for and about the patient in a much truer way.

Once hospice is suggested, the caregiver has to reorient her thinking. Suddenly, she must realize all over again that, in fact, this person is going to die – soon. The hospice team can be a crucial help at this point. They must be sensitive to the fact that this individual (or family) needs to start a new kind of grieving. The caregiver has lost touch with normal life and may not realize what her needs are. "Validate the fact that she is engulfed in pathological circumstances not of her own making. Such validation will help to relieve her sense of disenfranchisement and free her to grieve openly."[1] She needs to let go of the loved one and the caregiving experience. This will leave a major gap in her life. She can use much encouragement and discussion about what she will do with that time. When the hospice workers recognize that she has accepted the imminent nature of the death, it's time to help the caregiver start bringing back the past. They should ask about this patient, who he was, what he did, what he was like. Gradually, little by little, they can help the caregiver return to the place where she lost herself in the avalanche of this disease. She has lost the person her loved one was before. She has lost the social aspects of her former life. She has lost herself as spouse, daughter, sister, etc. When the loved one has died and the caregiving role is suddenly removed, there can be an overwhelming emotional vacuum. All the members of the hospice team can help minimize this by assisting the person to think through where she will go from here, where she was before Alzheimer's and how to put the pieces of her former life back together.

Also recognize the unique stresses that exist for the family in the nursing home setting. These are very specific needs that can be fulfilled by various members of the hospice team. The nursing home may employ one social worker for 100 patients or more. Little individual attention is given to the family. The family needs more attention in the end stages and nursing home staff is stretched to their maximum as it is. For an older spouse or family member, driving, shopping and visiting are all greatly appreciated.

If this patient has been in a facility for quite a length of time, empathize with staff too. They become like family members and will be grieving this loss as well. Ask them about the patient's life since residing in the nursing home. The night my mother died, three of the aides who had known her a long time stood with me around her bed and we talked about her. They all wanted remembrances of her which I gave them. They took the kite and rainbow from her ceiling and put them up in the dining room so "Bea will always be with us."

Patient Care

Hospice staff and volunteers who are not familiar with dementia patients may become frustrated by the seeming lack of response when using familiar skills. They may not give the patient credit for thoughts or feelings if they don't know how to recognize responses. As discussed in earlier chapters, caring for a patient based on his equivalent developmental age can be beneficial to the patient and to the hospice worker. Obviously, there are physical differences between an infant and the Alzheimer's patient, however, the patient and infant are equally vulnerable physically and emotionally.

The key thing to remember is that you must try to go where the patient is. You cannot get him to come to you. If he tells you he is standing on the street corner waiting for the trolley, that's where you go to meet him. You will not convince him that he is in the hallway of a nursing home. There are three probable states in which the hospice worker/volunteer will find Alzheimer's patients: still alert and talking; alert but not speaking; less responsive.

If he is still talking, ask him about his past – what kind of car did he drive; what kind of work did he do; how many people are in his family; where did they live, etc. If, at the time you are talking to him, he is back in time, go there and ask questions in the present tense. A person with Alzheimer's appreciates nothing so much as someone who acknowledges his reality. Trying to convince him of what is going on currently will only cause frustration and stress on his part and yours. Throw your reality out the window and affirm what he is feeling. You can do this without agreeing with him. Suppose you have a woman who tells you angrily that her husband is having an affair. She knows this is why he doesn't stay with her all the time. You could try just empathizing with her feelings. "It must be awfully frustrating to feel like he's not here enough." or "It must feel awful to think someone might do that." If you start out this way, the person is relieved at not being contradicted, pleased that someone seems to understand her feelings, and may then be willing to talk it out until you get her onto another subject or convince her (at least for the moment) that her husband loves her.

If his speech pattern is nonsensical, mirror for him the feelings he has. Assume his tone and expression so that he realizes you empathize with him. Recall that in Chapter I, I said that a person's emotional makeup does not diminish or change with dementia; neither does the need to be understood. There was one lady at the nursing home who was given to little spells of anger and/or distress. She couldn't speak intelligibly, but she would walk around grumbling, shaking her fist and gritting her teeth. Sometimes I would get right in her path and ask her what was wrong. She would grumble something and I would imitate the scowl on her face and say "That's terrible!" or "I guess I'd be angry too!" After a bit of this back and forth, the creases would gradually leave her face and she'd reach out smiling and stroke my face as if to say thank you for understanding. Another thing this particular lady responded to was music and dancing. If you took her hands and kind of swayed back and forth and hummed or sang, her whole demeanor would change. The one emotion you don't want to imitate is anxiety. If a person is very anxious or frightened, you need to respond with calm reassurance. Maintain a friendly facial expression and move carefully and deliberately so as not to startle him and throw him off balance.

If he is no longer speaking, but awake and alert most of the time, read to him or speak in soothing tones. Pray with/for him using prayers familiar to his religious background. You might want to collect a set of prayers to say for Jewish, Catholic, Protestant, Muslim persons. Show the person colorful pictures; pictures of pets, babies, cars, construction vehicles, flowers. Take him for a ride in a wheelchair, always moving slowly so that objects and people don't go by too quickly for him to take in. Consider a person walking by you, and as he passes, he touches you briefly, says "Hi!" and walks on, never stopping. You wouldn't think twice about that type of momentary greeting. Look at it, however, from the point of view of the Alzheimer's patient. A person with dementia needs time to process all incoming stimuli. A quickly moving person would make him anxious to begin with. A sudden touch may be startling, or at the very least, he would have to take time to realize what it was and who did it. The brief 'Hi' without stopping would be totally incomprehensible because of the movement and because he is still trying to interpret the touch on his shoulder.[2]

I often point out to my hospice classes the need to move slowly and deliberately with Alzheimer's patients because of their need to process information slowly. After one class with some Chaplains, I found out that one of them went to see a patient at a nursing home and was told that this person seemed quite agitated a lot of the time. The Chaplain went in and found that the head of the person's bed was by the door. Therefore, she never knew when someone was coming in. People would just sort of appear and start talking to her, or doing something for her, and it was too much for her to take in. The Chaplain suggested they turn the bed around so that she could see the doorway. They did, and it made all the difference.

For the patient who is even less responsive, keep in mind that the five senses are usually retained the longest. Appeal to his visual sense with bright colors, pictures (large enough to be seen if his vision is poor), baby dolls or stuffed animals. Satisfy his sense of hearing with music, old time radio programs, prayers, or just read to him. Often just the sound of someone's voice in the room gives a sense of security. Occasionally fill his room with the scent of flowers, coffee grounds, wood shavings, cologne. Give him something to hold in his hand like a small rubber ball or a rolled up washcloth, or something to wrap his arms around like a stuffed animal or a pillow. Massage him or brush his hair; wash his hands and face. A little caution with the sense of touch, however. Some patients can be hypersensitive to touch. Approach carefully and keep a respectful distance if he doesn't like being touched. The sense of taste may be dulled a bit with age and, at this stage, he may not be able to swallow well, but, if allowed, you could put tiny bits of mint or sugar or chocolate on his tongue just to give him the taste.

Once you have spent time with Alzheimer's patients, you begin to see that they do, indeed, respond to your presence and whatever you bring into their lives. It may be a smile, or shaking a finger at you, or grabbing your ID badge. It may be a deeper and more restful sleep as you sit by the bedside reading or playing music. It may be incoherent speech, but with a facial expression that tells you there is meaning there. You will undoubtedly miss these subtle signs if you are just passing by. You have to go where they are to 'hear' what they are trying to tell you.

An Alzheimer's patient cannot tell you what hurts, but you can see in his expression if something hurts when you try to move him or do mouth care, for instance. An Alzheimer's patient cannot ask you for special favors, but you'll know by his subtle responses when you have fulfilled his needs. An Alzheimer's patient cannot tell you about issues or relationships that need mending, but he may tell you what good things or painful things he is experiencing as a young man or child. (I read of an instance where a daughter found herself caregiver to a father with whom she didn't get along. As he regressed in time, he spoke with the greatest joy about his newborn baby girl. This was an unexpected healing for this father and daughter).

An Alzheimer's patient cannot prepare himself for death, but as his body gets weaker and his spirit gets stronger, getting ready to be free, I believe that for a brief time before the body dies, his spirit is very present to the family and hears and knows all that they are trying to tell him. This is a gift that you can give to the Alzheimer's family. Tell them that as their loved one nears the end of his life, he can hear them and he knows who they are.

*Portions of this chapter were originally published in the July/August 2002 issue of the American Journal of Hopsice and Palliative Care, Vol. 19, No. 4, pp 263-266.

[1] Dempsey, Marge RN BA, Baago, Sylvia MA (1998). Latent Grief: The Unique and Hidden Grief of Carers of Loved Ones With Dementia. In American Journal of Alzheimer's Disease. March/April

[2] Brackey, Jolene. (2003). Creating Moments of Joy, Enhanced Moments. Polk City. IA.

Chapter VI

For Police and Emergency Workers

When a person with Alzheimer's is involved in any type of crisis or emergency situation, the response of the police or other emergency personnel will be dramatically different than with any other type of encounter. The way in which the police officer interacts with this person will determine whether the incident will be brought under control fairly quickly or will amplify into a far more difficult situation. (For the sake of efficiency, I will refer throughout this chapter to police officers, but the majority of this information is also applicable to EMT's, firefighters, paramedics, emergency room personnel, etc.) What I will address here are the behaviors and signs of dementia to look for, the responses that will elicit cooperation, and how to handle difficult behaviors.

Behaviors

Odd behaviors come and go at the outset of this disease. Fluctuations in abilities may be inaccurately attributed to laziness, lack of concentration or unwillingness to cooperate. This all contributes to feelings of disbelief on the part of the individual and others. Take special note of the signs and symptoms so that when a true case of dementia is encountered, the individual can be treated with compassion. For instance, a person with Alzheimer's may be suspected as being drunk. However, on closer look, there will be no physical manifestations such as staggering, slurring of speech or alcoholic breath.

Early stages – signs/symptoms not easily recognized

- quite verbal and initially responds to questions sensibly, but sooner or later cannot answer properly (After some conversation you may realize that he thinks it's a different time or place).
- may know his name and address, but has no idea where he is or how he got there (gets lost in familiar places)
- may be stressed or anxious but doesn't know why; wringing hands, pacing, disjointed words (Anxiety stems from awareness of symptoms. He may avoid people so as to hide these symptoms).
- trouble retaining new information, recent conversations or events (Half an hour after detaining him, he doesn't recall your name or why he's with you).
- unable to follow instructions; cannot perform tasks with multiple steps
- 'poor historian' or seems odd
- defers to caregiver to answer questions if caregiver is present

Middle stages – signs/symptoms become more obvious

- repetitive statements and questions ('What time is it?' ' What is your name again?' Repetitive answers may be the only constant in his life).
- difficulty with words; difficulty following conversations
    may make up words/stories to fill in the blanks

    illogical speech

    cannot respond to simple questions

- disregard for rules of social conduct; inattentive to appearance; displays disturbing behaviors

    undressing in public

    questioning strangers

    unaware of danger (standing in road)

    unaware of environment (cold, darkness)

- passive and somewhat unresponsive
- unfocused or may be intensely focused on something
- irritable, suspicious (believes someone has stolen from him)
- may hallucinate (not harmful if it doesn't frighten him)
- functional difficulties under stress; perceptual-motor problems (getting in or out of car)
- purposeful wandering or searching behavior

First signs reported by persons with Alzheimer's –

    Take note if an individual describes any of these problems.

- cannot fully coordinate and control speech and actions
- loses track of conversations
- lost in familiar surroundings
- problem solving difficulties
- unable to concentrate; thought block; writing block
- inability to quickly recall names
- feeling disassociated from reality
- sadness, depression, feeling unduly angry

Responses

Keep in mind that all Alzheimer's patients are basically looking to communicate, to feel secure, and/or to be useful. If you consider their behaviors as stemming from one or more of these needs, it may be easier to understand and respond.

The other key is to go wherever he is. This is the same theme that I have repeated throughout this book, but it is significant for successful interactions. The person with Alzheimer's will not understand or respond to your reality. Especially in the middle and later stages, there is no logical, step-wise thinking. "If … then" thinking is beyond his capacity.

When you encounter someone whom you suspect may have some type of dementia, and he is alone, look for a "Safe Return,"[1] hospital or Wanderguard identification. A hospital or Wanderguard wrist or ankle bracelet will, obviously, tell you if this person has left a hospital or nursing home, and the nearest facilities can be contacted. "Safe Return" is a program sponsored by the Alzheimer's Association whereby families can sign up their loved one and provide them with a bracelet or necklace and iron-on clothing labels, with an 800 number on them. The person's information is kept on file and can be accessed readily so as to return the person safely home. (The caregiver can also obtain an identification bracelet so that if anything should happen to her, she will be identified as someone who provides care for a person registered with "Safe Return.") In your encounters with Alzheimer's families, if they are not already aware of this program, strongly suggest that they contact their local Alzheimer's Association and get their loved one signed up.

An early stage Alzheimer's person will be able to talk with you and may retain all the appropriate social skills. He may have a clear idea of who he is and possibly even where he lives, but as you converse with him, you will discover that he won't know where he is now or how he got there. You will need to accompany him home or to a hospital, whichever is appropriate, and make his family aware of this incident. This may be the earliest sign of Alzheimer's and the family may be unaware there is a problem as yet.

If he is carrying anything, ask, "Can you show me your wallet/pictures/purse?" This may help to identify him and/or may help him remember family members. It is more likely than not that he will trust you and be willing to show you whatever he has with him.

While attempting to determine his identification, you will want to use the following communication techniques:

- Approach slowly from the front. Speak only when visible to him. Tell him your name. Offer your hand – palm up and open. Smile and maintain a relaxed demeanor.

- Get on his level so that you can make eye contact and you don't appear threatening. A uniform makes you look taller and bigger.

- Stabilize any movement he makes. Trauma or stress can throw off his ability to function physically.

- If at all possible, talk to him alone. Too many people or voices will over stimulate and confuse him. If others are on the scene, move them or move the individual.

- Call him by name if you can find out what it is.

- Use few words, simple one thought questions or phrases.

- Repeat once or twice using the exact same words. If he still doesn't respond, then rephrase more simply.

- Give the person time to think and respond. He won't be quick to answer questions.

- Be literal. Sarcasm and cliches will not be understood.
- Use overemphasis, gestures, and point to objects. Different brain paths may be more alert than others.
- Offer concrete choices when questioning. Try multiple choice or yes/no questions. Open ended questions will throw him off and he won't be able to search out an answer. Also give direct instructions, not polite questions.

NOT HELPFUL	BETTER
Where are you coming from?	Are you coming from the store?
Where does it hurt?	Does it hurt here?
What do you want to drink?	Do you want water or Coke?
Do you want a drink?	Here's some water.
Would you like to come with me?	Come with me now.
Can you sit down?	Sit here. (and direct him)

If leading him by the hand doesn't work, sometimes body language will work. Beckon him to follow you if he doesn't want to be touched. Pictures or objects may trigger speech. Written words may be understandable. If the person is so anxious that he cannot follow the simplest of directions or words, try writing one-word directions. The ability to read is retained for some time. (i.e. Sit down. Come. Follow me. What is your name? I will help you).

He may think that he knows you. If so, go along with this. If he says it's nice to see you, ask how he's been since you last saw him. Come across as a friend and he will trust that you are one. People with Alzheimer's are often very trusting. This can be a danger for them, but in an emergency situation, it can be of real benefit to the person trying to help.

It's possible that your uniform may disturb him. If it does, try taking off your hat and sitting down with him. Always assume a friendly, non-official tone. Typically, however, the uniform will not be a concern. Most dementia patients I've seen react very favorably to anyone with a uniform and, in fact, interpret almost any type of uniform as police. We had one gentleman in the nursing home who would call out to maintenance men, service people, anyone in a dark outfit and ask them to arrest someone for him. Also, anyone in white or light clothing was "Doc."

Find and inform the family. This may initiate awareness and action by the family. They may not have been aware of a problem until some incident occurs, particularly if the individual lives alone and no one has monitored his behavior on a daily basis.

This individual needs to be kept from driving. As an authority figure, you may be able to convince him of this where the family has not been able to do so. Driving is one of the most difficult issues for an Alzheimer's family to face. It is often recommended that families turn to their family doctor, the Motor Vehicle Department or the police to intervene. Often, this type of official directive that a person cannot drive is accepted (not happily, but accepted) more easily than if it comes from a spouse or adult child. When a police officer or medical person steps into a situation where a person is lost or hurt, it may be just the right time to convince him that his safety is at risk.

The person in middle stages may be oblivious to any problem or may be quite anxious. He will be more likely to have language problems, and the more anxious he is, the less sense he will make. Assume his expression and tone. This reassures him that you understand. A person will calm down if he thinks you know how he feels. Mirror whatever emotion he is feeling except fear or anxiety. If he is fearful, be reassuring that you are going to help him.

If you can't understand what he is trying to tell you, watch his body language for clues, or look around him to see what he may be referring to. For instance he may be making hand motions that suggest what he is thinking or he may be looking in a specific direction. Try to pick out significant words from his nonsensical speech and respond to those. For example, if he uses the word 'boat' or 'train' or 'car,' ask if he's traveling somewhere. If he points at a sign, ask if he's looking for a particular street.

If the person is determined to go somewhere – Church, store, work, etc. – offer to take him there, but "first could we stop by the police station/my office/your house?" If he keeps asking about this place, ask him about it. Where is it; what do you need there; do you go there often; do you like it there; who is there, etc. You may change his focus and/or get useful information. Often times, just getting him in a car and driving around or walking him a bit may be enough to cause him to forget what his goal was.

A person with dementia cannot think in logical sequence. "If … then" thinking has no place in his mind. This is why he becomes anxious or suspicious. He knows something is wrong right now. There's something his mind cannot get hold of. He can't remember the past and there is no future; there is only now. You cannot reason with him by saying, "It's dark out. The store is closed." Pointing out why something cannot possibly be the way he perceives it will not register at all. Recall from Chapter I that a person loses his judgement and ability to see the consequences of his actions. When he gets it in his mind that he needs to do something, he will not stop and think, "It's cold outside. I'll freeze if I go out without a coat." He just goes. He will hide money in a box in the back of his closet and then claim it was stolen. He won't recall having done this before and he won't be able to reason that no one would have had the opportunity to steal it. An injured man in an emergency room will not realize that if he gets up and tries to walk away, he will make his injury worse.

Once again, you need to go where they are. Why are they behaving or reacting the way they are? Why are they stressed, angry, restless? If you know, adjust their environment. If you don't know, just go with them – "That must make you very angry!" "Oh, I'm sorry you're so sad." "Let's walk for a while."

Difficult Behaviors and Crises

In emergency situations (accident, fire, caregiver illness), the person with Alzheimer's will be pushed out into left field. Here, more than any other time, if at all possible separate the individual from the scene. If a family member or friend is available and is calm, have them do it. Reduce the number of people, sights and sounds as much as possible.

Unless it is necessary for safety, don't use force to resolve the situation. A person with Alzheimer's will take his cues from you, from your tone and behavior. Interact with him in a quiet, calm manner. If he trusts you, lead him away by the hand or by motioning for him to follow you. Leave him in the care of someone who can stay with him until the emergency situation is resolved. Do not ever leave him alone.

If the demented person is the victim, again, have one EMT, fire fighter or police officer tend to him. Find out his name or nick name if you can and use it frequently to reassure him you are a friend. Do you carry stuffed animals, playing cards, candy, etc. in your vehicle? These can be used to distract and comfort him.

Recognize the environmental stressors that may trigger more extreme behavior. Unfortunately, in an emergency situation, it's likely that all of these elements will be present.

- unfamiliar place
- too many sounds
- too loud a sound
- bright/flashing lights
- no familiar faces
- people moving too fast

Try to put yourself in his place. Reduce incoming stimuli as much as possible and you may prevent the situation from getting out of control beforehand.

Violence

Resistance, confrontation and violence are ways of communicating. The person is looking for something we are not providing. The first attempts at calming the person should be to provide that 'something' rather than use physical force against him. In an emergency, the cause of his violence might be obvious and to whatever extent is possible, change his situation accordingly.

For instance, if there is a fire, (and he is not injured) walk him or drive him as far away from the scene as possible, reassuring him that the fire has been put out and everything is fine now. Or if you encounter a man reacting violently toward his wife who is trying to get him to come back home, try to calm the caregiver and separate her momentarily, get the man's attention and try the questioning technique: Where are you going? What do you need there? Who will be there? Can I take you?

Someone in an emergency room, particularly if they don't see anyone familiar, may become frightened and aggressive. First of all, an aggressive episode may be avoided to begin with by making sure the individual is not left alone, by speaking to him calmly, by distracting him with pictures, conversation or food, and by taking him out in a wheelchair if treatment needs to be delayed. Walk him around outside or in the halls just to distract him from the idea of being confined and to take a break from the sights and sounds of a busy emergency room. When the clinician does come to treat him, she should sit down with him and chat with him briefly as a friend. Once she has his attention and trust, she can begin her examination one step at a time, making sure to tell him what she is about to do and why. He may not understand all that she is saying, but he will understand enough to go along as long as she doesn't rush and just start 'doing things' to him. (See Chapter III) Even though you may feel as though you can't take the time to stop and visit with the patient, consider it a worthwhile investment of time when you realize that you are probably avoiding a violent reaction and the need to call in three or four other people to hold the patient down while you finish your exam or treatment.

Again, try every means to find the cause of a violent outburst. If you can pinpoint that, change or eliminate it. Sometimes a firm "What do you want!?" will be just startling enough to get his attention and stop the episode momentarily. Then you quickly move in with calm questioning: What has made you angry? How can I help you? How can we fix this?

If the cause cannot be determined, one person should stay with the individual while others move people and objects out of harm's way. Try distraction techniques to relocate the person to a calmer, quieter environment. Experiment with diversions – music, food, exercise. Maybe this person is territorial and you are getting in his space. Maybe he doesn't like being led, but will follow you if you beckon without touching him. He may take an unexplained dislike to a particular person. If someone else is available, have him try to calm the individual and you step out of the picture. (If this works, by the way, don't assume it was your appearance or manner that generated the episode. It is most likely some obscure connection the person has made between you and someone he doesn't like).

Reduce aggression by improving the person's sense of safety, physical comfort and control. Make sure he knows you are trying to help him. Check as best you can for any physical injuries. Ask for his help in some small way. This will give him a sense that he has some control over the situation. Ask him to hold something for you, or sort or count something, or give him a notebook and ask him to make notes about the event.

Yelling/Wandering

See Chapter III on Difficult Behaviors for extensive coverage of these behaviors. If you encounter either of these behaviors in a person who is in your charge temporarily, you obviously cannot go looking for causes and behavior patterns from his past. The only thing to be concerned about is dealing with it in the short term.

The simplest and most effective solution is to get him moving if possible. Get him to walk around for exercise. This can be very relaxing for a person under stress. Accompany the person as he paces.

Give him something to do – folding, sorting, fixing something; or something to hold onto – a stuffed animal, tools, the packaging from bandages you are applying. Have simple toys, cards, poker chips or such on hand, or things that can be taken apart and reassembled fairly easily. Distract with food or ask him to perform some task for you.

Your purpose in the short term is to circumvent the person's wandering and to get him to stop yelling. On the other hand, if the yelling isn't bothering anyone, let him do it.

Police Encounters

What are some of the typical situations in which police will encounter people with Alzheimer's?

- wanderers – you discover a lost person or a caregiver calls to report a missing person
- shoplifters – individual unknowingly takes something and the store security may or may not realize this is a dementia case
- indecent exposure calls – remember, social graces are no longer intact
- you are called by the person with Alzheimer's about a theft
- an erratic driver

Possible scenarios and discussion of police encounters are found in Appendix B. Emergency room situations are presented in Appendix C.

---

[1] Safe Return. (1998). Alzheimer's Disease and Related Disorders Association, Inc.

Chapter VII

Spiritual Care

"In Thy book were written, every one of them, the days that were formed for me, when as yet there was none of them." (Ps 139:16) Every aspect of our lives has been seen by God before we ever were. His plan for some of us will include Alzheimer's; and for others, ministering to those with Alzheimer's. We can praise and thank God in advance for favors and graces we have not received yet. The psalmists do this frequently. Perhaps someone has thanked God for the grace of your assistance before he lost his ability to comprehend.

I won't repeat what has gone before, but refer to Chapter VI on Police and Emergency Workers for a list of the typical behaviors observed in the early and middle stages of Alzheimer's. In the end stages, which the pastoral care person will frequently encounter, the individual will have lost most of his physical functions. He will be incontinent, unable to walk, eventually will lose eye/hand coordination, will not be able to sit without support or hold his head up, and at the very end, will not be able to swallow. His ability to eat and swallow properly will regress from solid foods to ground foods to pureed foods to thickened liquids. He will startle easily and require total hands-on care. I have read that a person also loses the ability to smile, however, I have not seen this happen either in my mother or any other dementia patients I have been with in the final stages of this disease.

I will reiterate briefly some of the communication skills to be used with dementia patients, but see Chapter II and Chapter III for a more thorough coverage of these techniques.

Early stage persons will be able to talk with you. When he is able (some days are better than others), it can be beneficial to help him recall his history. Tape his reminiscences or write them down if he would like you to. This can give him a great deal of satisfaction and could be a gift to the family.

Remember to find out if you can, who he was before and then go where he is now. If he recognizes that you are there in a pastoral care role, it may take him back to an earlier Church or religious setting. Help him to enjoy that previous experience.

Basic strategies:

- approach slowly from the front; speak only when visible to him
- get on eye level with him
- support and stabilize any movement he makes
- use few words; simple one thought questions/phrases
- repeat exactly once or twice, then, if he still doesn't respond, repeat more simply
- give him time to think and respond

Pictures or objects may trigger speech. Ask about objects in his room or anything he is holding. "Can you show me your pictures?" If you can't understand what he is trying to tell you, watch his body language for clues or look around him to see what he might be referring to.

He may think he knows you. If so, go along with this. It will make communication easier. Go where he is. Recall that when he is 'somewhere else' he has no ability to think logically or sequentially. 'If ... then' thinking is beyond his capability.

Question him about where he is, what it's like, what he is doing. If he is unable to communicate clearly, assume his expression and tone to let him know you appreciate how he feels. If you are new in this person's life, it may be easier for you to interact with him in some respects than it is for family members. You have no knowledge of him previously and, therefore, can accept him for who he is and where he is now. The family may still be struggling with the loss of his (and their) former life. They may be so bogged down in caregiving and living the day to day experience, that creativity is not even a consideration. If they are open to it, assist them in finding ways to communicate with their loved one.

If he sees something you don't, go along with it. Illusions and hallucinations are harmless as long as they are not frightening.

Responding to the person based on an equivalent developmental age becomes more significant in the later stages of this disease. These are the comfort care stages. I recall an incident that touches my heart every time I think of it. I took my mother to Church one day and we entered through the attached school. Halfway down the hallway, our pastor, Fr. Robert Hale, was bending over, talking to a small child, admiring something she had in her hand. My mother hurried up to him and said, "Look! See what I have!" and showed him her rosary. Without so much as raising an eyebrow, he turned to her and said, "Oh, yes. That's lovely too!" and fussed over her just as he had the little girl. I don't know if he was aware at the time that she had Alzheimer's, but in the instant that it took him to assess the situation, he responded more graciously than most people we encountered throughout the length of her disease. And trust me when I tell you, an act of kindness like this does more to bolster the caregiver than it does the patient. We both walked into Church with a lighter step.

In the end stages, keep in mind that the five senses are the doors of communication. Appeal to sight, sound, scent, touch and taste.

Always be aware of the value of life. Love is not just giving, but receiving. This person is the ultimate receiver of love. He has a soul and a soul is not just who we are and what we do, but what God acts upon. God is surely acting upon this person's life and is bringing him into your life for a reason. A newborn has no memories, voice or physical capabilities, but we know he has a soul and a life worth living. So too with Alzheimer's. Just because the individual is not what we remember him to be or what we would like him to be, it doesn't automatically follow that his life is worthless. Look at the people who come into his life after Alzheimer's. Watch how they relate to him. They don't see him as pathetic, incapable of communication. Encourage your families to watch for and treasure these types of reactions and to learn from them.

Ministering to the Individual

"Moral, devotional and spiritual aspects of life are crucial for the full, rich life of the soul. The soul is 'self' AND that which God acts on. Some link the soul more with our consciousness than with God's work within us. This leaves little room for grace and it is difficult to see then how God can be present in and vitalize a person with Alzheimer's."[1]

"Each human life consists of a story that began before that person was aware of it and therefore presumably can continue after he or she again ceases to be aware of it."[2]

The soul, spirit, core of one's being, needs to relate to the universe in which it lives via emotional, religious, social, physical, and mental routes until death. My value is measured by the interaction of my life with others and with God. Aging breaks down physical and mental capacities. Dementia distorts all five functions. However, the core remains whole. Those experiences which by repetition and value have become a part of the core remain whole. Singing hymns, reciting prayers no longer seem to be the function of mind or memory, but distinctly spiritual.[3] The key is learning a person's spiritual history.

A person is identified by being called by name. When one is losing identity, his name brings it back. Hearing one's name touches his spirit.

Touch is our most intimate, powerful and positive form of communication. A simple touch can reduce the heart rate and lower blood pressure. It can reduce physical and psychological pain, relieve anxiety, diffuse anger and build self-esteem. We can offer non-threatening touch by walking hand in hand, by a handshake, admiring jewelry, brushing one's hair or lightly massaging the back or shoulders.

People with dementia cannot initiate activities to help fulfill spiritual needs, but they may maintain a deep desire for spiritual fulfillment. Needs can be fulfilled by the simplest acts of kindness.

- Enable the person to continue attending religious services as long as possible.
- Continue religious practices for those who cannot do it themselves; prayer, scripture, hymns.
- Keep in mind you are not trying to engage his intellectual capacities. Do not attempt to introduce something new into his life.

Religious books or booklets with biblical pictures may give pleasure. Music familiar to childhood touches the heart and soul as well as the mind.

Scripture should be a familiar version; for instance the King James Version for Protestants or Douay-Rheims or Ignatius Bible for Catholics.

Religious objects or symbols help a person know where he is and what is expected. A person with dementia responds to faith rituals and symbolism. He may not know where he lives or what day of the week it is, but he may very well respond to the colors of the vestments and altar cloths in the Church. If he sees the pastor wearing purple, he automatically realizes that it must be Lent. Some of the symbols that may be significant:

holy water	statues	candles	menorah
wine	rosary	incense	Star of David
vestments	cross/crucifix	prayer books	Communion host
Latin	Hebrew	medals	scapular

Encourage a sense of security, comfort and familiarity. The person should not feel vulnerable to his own confusion, and therefore wonder if God still loves him. At the 1998 Alzheimer's national conference, Rev. Arlan Menninga told of a Protestant minister with Alzheimer's who had been placed in a nursing home. His family reported that he hardly spoke at all and they feared he had forgotten his faith. However, one day when he was brought to a prayer service at the nursing home, part way through the service, he stood up and asked to speak. He was warmly invited to do so and came up to the pulpit and gave a 'sermon.' Not all of it was intelligible, but he was clearly in his element. Given the appropriate setting, he knew his role.

After wrestling for weeks with the frightening feeling that his relationship with Christ was gone, Robert Davis wrote, "As I lay in a motel crying out to my Lord, my long desperate prayers were suddenly answered. The sweet, holy presence of Christ came to me. He spoke to my spirit and said, 'Take my peace. Stop your struggling. It's all right. This is all in keeping with My will for your life. I now release you from the burden of the heavy yoke of pastoring that I placed upon you. I will hold you. Lie back in your Shepherd's arms and take My peace.'"[4]

Now certainly, for most people, a sense of their place in God's plan won't come as dramatically as it did for Rev. Davis. That is why we must provide this sense of God's peace and love for them. By holding religious services for dementia patients, we let them know they are not alone and that they still have a place in corporate worship.

Encourage a sense of self-worth. Convey the message that he is worth the attention, care and time given to him. Assure him that he does things well. Have him retell stories. Rev. Davis also wrote, "I fear the day when my mind will lose this capacity to know God's love. Then I must rely solely on those who love me to keep me close to the Father by their prayers, songs, touch and words of Scripture."[4]

Some ideas for nurturing a person's spirit are to help them find joy in God's creation. Walk outdoors or watch National Geographic TV shows. Record the Bible on tape; preferably have a familiar voice read it. Davis suggests a 'Promise Box,' that is, cards with a Bible verse for each day of the year. And listen to the person's concerns about losses and grief in the early stages of Alzheimer's disease. This can help him work through feelings of sadness and anger, even at God. His perception of loss and fear must be accepted as real.

Group Religious Activities

Offer people with Alzheimer's Disease the opportunity to express their faith often. They cannot remember the last service, nor can they anticipate the next. Now is all there is.

The whole service need not be brief, but each part should be. A possible outline of a prayer service could include:

- hymns (one verse each)
- short prayers (regarding family, aging, loneliness)
- 2 readings (regarding hope and encouragement)
- 3-5 minute sermon (stories from your personal experience; the Alzheimer's patient is looking for ways to connect with other human beings; focus on relationships rather than on abstract ideas)
- Lord's Prayer
- a blessing which offers peace and encouragement

Keep the service simple with only one thing going on at a time. Sometimes trying to lead them with a voice and a piano can be confusing. Unless it is a well-known prayer or reading such as the Lord's Prayer, group readings may not work. It takes too many thought processes to read from a book, hear others' voices, and try to pace oneself with others. Don't try to teach new hymns or prayers. You must go back to what was familiar when they were growing up in their faith. This will reawaken their spirituality. Also, make the setting familiar. For instance, if you set the chairs in a circle, they will have no idea what they are there for. Set chairs and lectern, etc. as they would be in a Church or Temple setting. Obviously, the setting must also be inviting to wheelchairs, walkers and canes.[5]

Music should be familiar to the participants' childhood experiences. It may take some doing to find the right music. I had to search long and hard to find some tapes of Catholic music that would have been familiar to my mother. The vast majority of tapes out there had modern hymns and music on them; they were lovely, but totally foreign to her. I finally found three tapes with older Catholic hymns – which had music and words – and I found a tape of a Latin Mass in Gregorian Chant.

Other religious devotionals which may spark a memory;

May Crowning of the Blessed Virgin	Corpus Christi procession
Christmas/Easter liturgies	Passover/Yom Kippur
gathering a minyan for mourners	Kaddish
Stations of the Cross	

Ministering to the Caregiver

When Jesus chastised His disciples for criticizing the woman anointing His feet, He temporarily gave second place to His commandments about giving to the poor. A loving act of caregiving to One so close to torture and death transcended financial concerns. Jesus goes on to say that "what she has done will be told in memory of her." The beauty of faithful caregiving evokes history. "Caregivers may be living embodiments of the Kingdom which was established by a crucified Lord, not a Davidic king. Love given as crosses are taken up foreshadows a time when we all may be able to love without concern for our own wants."[6]

A caregiver loses a sense of her history with the patient and measures her caregiving according to her own memories. Her memories may bring comfort and continuity, but without being able to share the memories of the other, a bond is broken. She must be encouraged to put her memories on hold. Until we can put our memories on a back burner, pack them up and put them away – for now – we cannot live in the here and now with our loved one. We continue to live in the past without him or her.

A caregiver loses a sense of who she is. There is no 'I' in the act of caring, but rather 'I must' be true to others. As ministers you must reaffirm her selflessness. Reassure her that she is not giving up or losing the best part of her life for nothing, but rather that she is showing forth the best that she is in giving her life for another. It is not a part of her life lost, but a part of her life she will never regret.

You must encourage her in her faith. She must have faith that there is meaning in this activity, that she is learning, and that ultimately she will see that she has done the good thing. ("He has showed you what is good; and what does the Lord require of you but to do justice, and to love kindness and to walk humbly with your God." [Mic 6:8]) She must entrust herself and her loved one to God and know this is somehow a part of His plan.

To come full circle in caregiving, the caregiver must have an awareness of finality. She must have a perception of sacredness and sacramental acts. All things are redeemed in time. She will appreciate 'contemplative' visits when the loved one has moved beyond responsiveness. "Enduring is truer than withholding." When the realization of finality exists, there is a different kind of presence.[7]

These are four aspects of caregiving that you should bring to light for the caregiver: memory, authenticity, faith and finality. Assist the caregiver to think through these things, determine how they might apply to her, and through them to recognize the significance of the task of caregiving.

There are so many examples throughout Scripture which address the issues of suffering, consolation, caregiving, forgetting and remembering. The caregiver can identify with these and express her struggle:

"Then Samson called to the Lord and said, 'O Lord God, remember me I pray Thee, and strengthen me.'" (Jdg 16:28)

"Yet does not one in a heap of ruins stretch out his hand and in his disaster cry for help?" (Job 30:24)

"Why hast Thou forgotten me?" (Ps 42:9)

"Let my prayer come before Thee, incline Thy ear to my cry! For my soul is full of troubles." (Ps 88:2-3)

"...and if children, then fellow heirs with Christ, provided we suffer with Him in order that we may also be glorified with Him." (Rom 8:17)

She can also receive consolation:

"When he calls to Me, I will answer him; I will be with him in trouble; I will rescue him and honor him." (Ps 91:15)

"I will trust and will not be afraid; for the Lord God is my strength and my song." (Is 12:2)

"For it is the God Who said, 'Let light shine out of darkness,' who has shone in our hearts." (2Cor 4:6)

"Though our outer nature is wasting away, our inner nature is being renewed every day. For this slight momentary affliction is preparing us for an eternal weight of glory beyond all comparison." (2Cor 4:16-17)

Over and over, God shows He is pleased with caregivers:

"Do not shrink from visiting a sick man, because for such deeds you will be loved." (Sir 7:35)

"...if you pour yourself out for the hungry and satisfy the desire of the afflicted, then shall your light rise in the darkness..." (Is 58:10)

"Whoever gives to one of these little ones even a cup of cold water ... truly, I say to you, he shall not lose his reward." (Mt 10:42)

"For God is not so unjust as to overlook your work and the love you showed for His sake in serving the saints as you still do." (Heb 6:10)

The caregiver can ask God to remember for the loved one:

"Then God remembered Rachel and God hearkened to her..." (Gen 30:22)

"Samson called to the Lord and said, 'O Lord remember me I pray Thee and strengthen me." (Jdg 16:28)

"I formed you; you are my servant, O Israel; you will not be forgotten by Me." (Is 44:21)

God knows what it is to forget and be forgotten. He can forget, but only to our benefit:

"...for I will forgive their iniquity, and I will remember their sin no more." (Jer 31:34)

God feels the separation from His people when we forget Him:

"Remember also your Creator ... before the years draw nigh when you will say, 'I have no pleasure in them.'" (Eccl 12:1)

"When they had fed to the full and were filled, and their heart was lifted up, therefore, they forgot Me." (Hos 13:6)

Finally, on the Cross, having taken on all the sins of mankind, a veil temporarily descends between Jesus and the Father, and Jesus cries out:

"My God, My God, why hast Thou forsaken Me?" (Ps 22:1)

At the same time, He knows that in hearing the first line of this Psalm, those nearby would automatically bring to mind the whole of it including –

"For He has not despised the affliction of the afflicted; and He has not hid His face from him but has heard when he cried to Him.

"All the ends of the earth shall remember and turn to the Lord.

"... and proclaim His deliverance to a people yet unborn."

"When God remembers us, then, He also remembers being forgotten Himself, a terrifying abandonment for which we sinners all share responsibility. We may wonder, perhaps, if His own experience on the Cross facilitates His remembering of Alzheimer's patients in nursing homes."[10]

Do we feel rewarded and compensated for the love and worship we offer to God? Not necessarily. We do these things because they are right. By the same token, while we don't feel rewarded by an unresponsive dementia patient, we show him love and devotion because it is right. Tell the caregiver, as often as she needs to hear it, she will 'feel' in eternity what she 'knew' in time.

In the book of Job we are told that Job's friends sat with him in silence for seven days and nights before they said a word. I heard it said that sitting on an ash heap with a friend for a week should entitle one to say just about anything he wants afterward. But another writer refers to this event in this way: "The friends sitting in silence paid attention to the 'survival' level of suffering, that is, God's presence with the sufferer through the friends. When they moved to theologizing, they dealt with Job's suffering on the intellectual level, which was much easier for them, but which distanced Job and the friends from God's presence in Job's suffering."[8] The caregiver can identify with the 'silent' friends, allowing God's presence to be felt with herself and her loved one; also the one who ministers to the caregiver should see him or herself in the person of the silent friends.

What about the caregivers with the questions; 'Why does God allow this to happen?' or 'Why him?' or 'Why me?' More to the point, why not. Beyond all the things in life about which we are not sure, the one thing we cannot doubt is that God knows what it is to suffer. He has been there. He has suffered to a greater extent than any one of us could ever imagine or experience. When we suffer, He is right in the midst of that suffering with us. Why should we be spared when He Himself wasn't. "Instead of explaining our suffering, God shares it."[9] Our late Holy Father, John Paul II, when asked if he might retire because of his sufferings, replied, "Jesus didn't get off the Cross. Neither will I." Clearly, he knew the redemptive value of suffering.

Contributions by the Faith Community

The faith community can share the burden of Alzheimer's families. They can, in the process, discover the meaning and value in suffering and recognize the right to continuation of life. They most certainly should maintain a spiritual connection with these families. The community can be humbled by the love and giving of caregivers. We may all need inspiration from dedicated caregivers.

"As the community accepts the responsibility of believing for a newly baptized infant, so too at the end of life does the Church accept this task for those in end stage dementia."[10]

What can the faith community learn about and offer?

- knowledge of community resources
- faith based support groups
- religious care facilities
- appropriate worship services
- coping styles of patients and caregivers

- respite care so the caregiver can attend Bible studies or other Church functions
- learn life stories of the patients

A committee can be formed to prepare and provide 'reminiscent packets' to nursing homes. These are packets that visitors can use to facilitate their visits with the Alzheimer's patient. It may encourage those who might not otherwise visit because they don't know what to do or say.

One's faith background may be forgotten or neglected in a skilled nursing facility. Residents are unable to fully participate in religious services and activities. Slowly their spiritual life fades away. Packets can rekindle the light. Here are some starter ideas.

For a Protestant resident:

Bible (King James Version)	Cross	pictures of Jesus
Companion of Prayer	Lord's Prayer	23rd Psalm
Ten Commandments	Apostles Creed	

For a Jewish resident:

Prayer book	Yarmulkes (2)	Prayer shawls (2)
Tefillin	Mezuzah	Candlesticks

For a Catholic resident:

Crucifix	Rosary	Scapular
Sacred Heart Badge	Statue of Mary	Catholic prayers
Lord's Prayer	23rd Psalm	10 Commandments
Apostles Creed	Hail Mary	Magnificat
Mysteries of the Rosary	Holy cards	Sacred Heart

You might also want to bring one or two little items that you can leave with the resident, perhaps a prayer card or cross, because he won't necessarily understand that he can't keep the items you are showing him from the packet.

Talk with the caregiver about how she feels the clergy might help the Alzheimer's person at worship services. Suggest that a sense of the familiar often cues appropriate behavior. Perhaps if the caregiver sits in a familiar spot or on the aisle, provides a rosary, prayer or hymn book, bulletin, brings snacks, religious cards, this will help. Also consider that the clergy person is in a good position to initiate talks with the family about the disease and to encourage a diagnostic work up. Like the police or doctor, a clergy person as a respected authority figure could discourage the individual from driving.

Suppose a person calls out during church services. The pastor could respond, "Bless you, John. We can all pray for each other." He calls on the congregation to lift John in prayer. Can you see how this incorporates the dementia patient into the worship service rather than to ignore him and leave his family with a sense of embarrassment? When you pray for/with him, you recognize his pain, his strength of perseverance, refocus his personal fears and respond with grace.

Clergy can model comfort and acceptance during worship if behavior is not appropriate. If John wanders up and down the aisle, the pastor could reach out his hand and invite him to stand or sit next to him, or he could just allow him to walk if it is not disruptive. Before the service, the congregation can welcome him, saying how glad they are to see him – but not several people at once. A parishioner can reassure him, "You are safe here with me," if he seems anxious. Volunteer to help the family and provide respite. Perhaps different members of the congregation can take turns walking him outside thereby allowing the family to stay through the entire service.

We mustn't assume that ministering to the person with Alzheimer's is strictly the job of the ordained clergy. We are all qualified to reach another's spirit from our own experience. Nor must we presume that this individual is beyond spiritual need. That which has been embedded into the core of his being from childhood has become a part of who he is and will be reachable in some way right to the end. Even if you find yourself sitting by the bedside of a totally unresponsive person and praying or reading scripture out loud, know that you are doing good. I heard of a hospice volunteer who did just that. She sat for several days with a comatose patient and prayed. As it turned out, this patient became somewhat alert before the end, and the first thing she asked was, "Where is the prayer lady?" You never know.

Some possible ministerial situations and discussions are presented in Appendix D.

[1] Keck, David (1996). Forgetting Whose We Are, Chapt. 4. Abingdon Press. Nashville.

[2] Sapp, Stephen (1997). "Memory: The Community Looks Backward," p50. In God Never Forgets. Ed. Donald K. McKim. Published bv Westminister John Knox Press.

[3] Menninga, Arlan. (1998). The Spiritual Care of Persons with Dementia. Presented at the Seventh Annual Alzheimer's Disease Education Conference. Indianapolis, IL.

[4] Davis, Robert (1989). My Journey Into Alzheimer's Disease, pp.55,110. Tyndale House Publishers, Inc. Wheaton, Illinois.

[5] Pohlman, Elizabeth. Eddy Alzheimer's Services, Troy, NY. Bloom, Gloria, Alzheimer's Assn. Capital District Chapter. Albany, NY 1992

[6] Keck, David (1996). Forgetting Whose We Are, p.216. Abingdon Press. Nashville.

[7] Bugbee, Henry. (1958). The Inward Morning. University of Georgia Press. Athens

[8] Simundson, Daniel (1980). Faith Under Fire: Biblical Interpretations of Suffering, p97. Augsburg. Minneapolis.

[9] Wolterstorff, Nicholas. (1987). Lament for a Son, p 81. Eerdmans. Grand Rapids.

[10] Keck, David (1996). Forgetting Whose We Are, pp 45-48, 91. Abingdon Press. Nashville.

Chapter VIII

Alzheimer's in the Workplace

How does corporate America deal with Alzheimer's – or do they? Here we will take a look at how businesses can address the employee with Alzheimer's, how an employer can assist the employee-caregiver, and how the employee-caregiver can work with his employer to do his best for both family and work.

Studies have shown that a large percentage (upwards of 25%) of American workers are balancing elder care and a full- or part-time job. Some caregivers quit their jobs, some will take a leave of absence and the majority will miss some work by coming in late or taking long lunches to deal with home responsibilities. Absenteeism and turnover could be costing American businesses millions of dollars per year.

There is a cost or financial loss for the caregivers as well: wage reductions, lost retirement benefits, lost assignments or promotions and health related problems.

Whether you look at this from a corporate or a personal perspective, the cost is unacceptable. Some corporations have added an elder care facet to their benefits package to entice workers; others have a crisis-oriented response. What can be done by and for businesses to cope with elder care issues?   What do employers and employees need and want to help circumvent or minimize these types of financial losses?

I looked at a whole list of surveys that have been done all over the country on work and family issues and found common outcomes reported:

- Workers who used company work-family benefits were absent less often than other workers.
- Informal work-family practices have a positive impact on worker's perceptions of their families which increases the organizational commitment of workers.
- Employees rate flexibility among the top five actions offered by management.
- The same innovative, systemic changes that ease work-life dilemmas will also help to achieve business goals.
- Most likely to be generous in the areas of work-life assistance are finance, insurance and real estate services. Least generous are wholesale and retail trades.
- Men said they would reduce their hours and salary by 18% to get more flexibility. Women said 23%. 76% said they would give up rapid career advancement for more flexibility.
- Operating expenses were cut through telecommuting and flexible work hours: higher productivity, fewer facilities, greater geographical hiring pools.
- Employees who use work-life programs are more likely to 'go the extra mile' to assure the success of the company.
- Employees reported that the ability to balance work with personal and family responsibilities had a positive impact on their decision to remain with the company.

- Workers with access to such benefits showed significantly more commitment to their employers.
- The more benefits workers use, the more they perceive the company as supportive and they, in turn, are supportive of the company.
- Employees who used the company's family supportive programs said these programs were a very important factor in their decision to stay with the company.

Clearly, working with the employee to accommodate his work and family needs benefits both the employee and the company. An employee who feels trusted and supported by management will give more to his job and maintain a higher level of loyalty to that company. The employer who feels that he is getting the best effort from his employee will be far more likely to allow flexibility in work hours.

Recognizing the Employee with Alzheimer's

While it is relatively uncommon for a person to be identified with Alzheimer's Disease on the job, it does happen. More often than not, this disease will manifest itself beyond retirement age, but early onset cases have been diagnosed while the person is still working. Management, indeed, all employees, should be aware of the signs and symptoms that might be noticed.

A review of Chapter I on the behaviors noted in the earlier stages of Alzheimer's Disease will give a good picture of the types of things that may stand out when someone you work with seems to be acting differently. A summary list of the early signs from Chapter VI is included here. A person in the early stages of this disease;

- is quite verbal and initially responds to questions sensibly, but sooner or later cannot answer properly,

- may know his name and address, but momentarily has no idea where he is or why he's there,

- may be stressed or anxious but doesn't know why; wringing hands, pacing, disjointed words,

- has trouble retaining new information, recent conversations or events,

- is unable to follow instructions; cannot perform tasks with multiple steps,

First signs reported by persons with Alzheimer's –

Take note if an individual describes any of these problems, even though you may not have noticed them yourself.

- cannot fully coordinate and control speech and actions
- loses track of conversations
- lost in familiar surroundings
- problem solving difficulties
- unable to concentrate; thought block; writing block
- inability to quickly recall names
- feeling disassociated from reality
- sadness, depression, feeling unduly angry

Assuming one or more of these problems have been observed, what is the first step in getting help for the individual? I would suggest if you are personal friends with the individual and his family, you might approach the family to find out if they have seen any similar behaviors, and to make them aware of what you have witnessed. Then, if your observations bear out, make Human Resources aware of the issues. If you are not personally associated with him or you are uncomfortable at the prospect of speaking to him or his family, you could go to Human Resources or his immediate supervisor with the information you have. If others in the work area have also reported problems, take note of their input and include this in reporting your observations HR.

An evaluation of the individual in his work setting needs to be done. A frank discussion of the issues should take place right away. If the individual is in the earliest stage of Alzheimer's and wants to – and is able to – continue working, certain accommodations should be made for him. The Americans with Disabilities Act states that some mental disabilities as well as physical disabilities require that the employer facilitate the work situation for the person in question. In the case of a person with Alzheimer's, he could be placed in a less complex job where fewer tasks and decisions need to be carried out. He should be given a work environment with few distractions so as to be able to focus on one task at a time. His work should be monitored and reviewed frequently with a positive, not an accusatory attitude. Supervisors need to reassure the person that they want to be helpful and enable him to work as long as he is able. If he feels like the supervisor is just looking over his shoulder for an excuse to get rid of him, this will add to his stress and increase mistakes. If an honest and open relationship is maintained between the employer and employee, it will be easier for both to recognize and accept when the employee can no longer work.

When continuing on the job is no longer an option, Human Resources needs to help him and his family with financial planning. A review of his current health benefits, qualification for disability insurance and/or early retirement benefits would be in order. Keep in mind that his family is starting down a very emotionally and financially stressful road and the more the company can come to their aid at the outset, the easier it will be for them.

Assisting the employee-caregiver

As noted earlier, nearly a quarter of employed Americans are trying to balance their work life and caregiving at home. This could range from simply running errands and handling finances up to complete care for activities of daily living. In some cases, caregivers report that working makes caregiving easier and less stressful. The job is an outlet and time away from the burdens of care. And, of course, caregivers who can afford to work a full-time job and pay for in-home care, day care or nursing home care experienced the least amount of stress. However, these families are the exception. Typically, the caregiver needs to work, cannot afford in-home care and, as a result, ends up cutting back on her hours, coming in late, taking longer lunches and spending more time on the phone trying to manage the home situation.

There are measures the employer can take to alleviate the stress of the caregiver and to gain the most productive hours while the employee is on the job, and Human Resource personnel need to be provided with the information they need to help employees. With the appropriate information, they can proactively work toward changing or improving company policies toward home and family issues.

The first and easiest thing for a company to provide is an informational clearing house for the types of services available to the employee in the community. Work is the one place you go every day. Making these references conveniently accessible in a 'one-stop' location can go a long way toward supporting the employee-caregiver. They should maintain a listing or handbook of sources for;

- geriatric management; agencies or individuals who provide assistance and coordination of services as needed

- homemakers and home health aides
- companion services
- respite care either in-home or in a facility to give caregiver time off (usually up to two weeks)
- home delivered meals
- legal assistance resources
- financial assistance resources
- Medicare/Medicaid information
- provide a listing of Internet sites for caregivers such as: http://www.caregiver.org/caregiver/jsp/home.jsp

http://aoa.gov

Just providing information on all these types of programs within your specific community can be a great relief for the caregiver who may not know how to start looking for help. Often times the caregiver gets so caught up in the day to day effort of caregiving and work and other family responsibilities, she may not even be aware that so many community resources are available. Pulling it altogether for her can save much time phoning and searching on her own.

Next, how can the employer directly assist the employee-caregiver? Here are some options that have been tried by various companies.

- Conduct a needs survey to determine what the level of interest is for assistance with elder care issues.
- Educate through seminars, presentations, articles in company newsletter on elder care practices.
- Offer support groups or counseling.
- Offer long-term care insurance.
- Reimburse or subsidize visiting nurse services.

- Elder Care Pager Program providing employee with a pager, free of charge, as long as they have need of it.
- Flexible scheduling, alternative work hours, compressed work weeks
- Job sharing, part-time employment
- Telecommuting
- Leave of absence
- Provide or find transportation for elders.

Surveys have shown time and again that any type of supportive gesture by management goes a long way toward motivating the employee to give her best effort on the job. The employee-caregiver who is stretched to capacity at home and at work is impeded by the actual tasks of caregiving, but also by the stress of trying to keep up with all her responsibilities and feeling like she is doing it all alone. Then, too, there is the very real result of stress related health problems for the caregiver causing more lost work hours. Just relieving the stress of this balancing act also reduces the burden, and all aspects of the caregiver's life improve. When the employer provides support, information and flexibility, everybody wins.

Finally, for the supervisors and co-workers directly involved with the employee-caregiver, recognize that this individual especially needs to feel your support. The attitude of the immediate supervisor is very important in influencing whether or not an individual takes advantage of the benefits available. Even though a benefit may exist on paper, managers may send mixed signals if employees try to use the benefit and they feel a sense of disapproval – another source of stress on an already burdened employee.

Ideally, the supervisor should be very positive about arranging alternative work hours or other types of assistance. He and the co-workers should be aware that the caregiver will have good days and bad days and try to tune in to her current stress level. Be patient with occasional flare-ups. Ask about the family member and allow the person to tell you what is going on at home – as many times as she needs to. Keep in mind that with Alzheimer's, not only is the person undergoing the stress of work and caregiving and all that goes with it, but she is also experiencing a grieving process as she loses the loved one little by little. The supervisor can reassign more difficult projects temporarily and try to avoid assigning tight deadlines. My boss used to do this for me, and periodically we would sit down, reassess my priorities and he would spread out the work, if necessary, among the other people in the lab. One of the nicest things the group did for me was when I took a personal day. I had to take my mother to a doctor's appointment that afternoon, but I decided to take the whole day off and get some time for myself in the morning. I left the house at the usual time, went and had breakfast at a restaurant, shopped, went to the library and by the time I got home, Mom was contentedly waiting for me. It turns out, one thing I hadn't thought of was that she called the lab on a regular basis with one crisis or another. All my co-workers knew what my plans were and that morning, when she called, they told her I couldn't come to the phone because I was working very hard but that I'd be home at noon. They kept her calm all morning.

If you haven't been there, you can't imagine what just a little encouragement and support can do. Management has the capacity to provide so much more than 'a little' support, and if they do, the employee-caregiver will pay them back with far more productive work hours, less time off, and long term loyalty.

The Employee-Caregiver's Role

The employee-caregiver must be up front with her supervisor. When an employee starts missing work, coming in late, being distracted on the job without explanation, the work environment becomes difficult for everyone; employee, supervisor and co-workers. Eventually the supervisor has no option but to take disciplinary action. However, if the employee explains her situation, the stresses she is experiencing, her needs both at work and at home and her limitations, it provides the supervisor with the opportunity to work out some sort of compromise. It tells management that you are willing and anxious to do a good job, and if flexibility is allowed, you will continue to be productive in your job.

Ideally, this conversation will take place before the stresses of caregiving have taken their toll. You must be realistic about the progression of caregiving. It won't always be just a matter of running a few errands. Eventually, the loved one will need more and more assistance and supervision. Perhaps he will come to live in your home which will initially save you worry and the need to run between two houses, but it will evolve into 24-hour-a-day needs. You may, in time, hire in-home assistance, but the paid caregiver will be calling you at work with problems and issues that need to be resolved. Your loved one may become total hands-on care during your off-work hours. You will be stretched financially, socially and emotionally. Before all this occurs, you need to anticipate the needs you will have with regard to your work responsibilities.

If you are realistic early in the caregiving process, you can have a reasonable discussion with management regarding what sort of assistance or flexibility you will need. You need to clarify your needs for yourself as well as your boss. Suggest a compromise such that your employer can see you intend to give the best to your job as well as your home life. Also leave the door open to further negotiation as your circumstances change. If you wait until you have reached a crisis point, it will no longer be a reasonable discussion, but rather a meeting of desperation calling for immediate, drastic change.

Some of the options that might be considered are

- later or earlier hours
- longer lunch time
- job sharing
- spontaneous time off to be made up within a day or two
- part-time hours

If a flexible schedule can be worked out between you and your boss, do your best to focus on work when at work. Your supervisor will be more willing to compromise if you have a track record of an excellent work ethic previous to this situation, and if you prove yourself dependable from this point forward.

Also take advantage of any references your company has to community resources. If your company has some type of employee assistance program, you can use them for counseling and advice as well as a source for eldercare issues.

There are four possible care options that you as employee-caregiver will be dealing with. First is that your loved one is home alone while you are at work, either in his own home or yours. In this instance, you will want to encourage friends or relatives to visit often. Ask neighbors to look in or at least keep an eye on the house to make sure he isn't leaving. Remove knobs from the stove and take all guns out of the house. Get a post office box if the mail makes him nervous or if he takes and hides it. Leave 'projects' for him to do – sewing, folding, writing, cleaning, yard work. Unless it is an acceptable situation in your particular job, it is best that he not have your work number. The calls will become more and more frequent. Rather, you should call him once or twice a day, when time allows. On the other hand, if the ringing phone upsets him, you may want to get an answering machine and turn the phone off when you are not there. The 'home alone' option is always the most worrisome, but in many cases, there is no other option. Your loved one may be at an early enough stage of the disease to refuse help of any kind. You and he may be financially limited as to what you can do. The best you can do is to make every effort to make sure he is safe. Stop home during lunch time, if possible. Make sure he doesn't have a workable car available. (You might leave him the keys, but disable the car).

A second scenario is to have in-home care in the form of a companion, assistant or aide. This is a far more comfortable idea, but, private help can be difficult to find and if you have one person on whom you depend, there is no backup if he or she is not available. Going through an agency doesn't always guarantee reliability. Either you have one regular aide who periodically can't be there, or you have different aides all the time which can be very confusing to the Alzheimer's patient. However, if you can find good, consistent in-home care, this is a situation that gives you more confidence and less worry at work. I happened onto a great system with my Mother when we reached this level of care. I found two women, cousins, who alternated days and filled in for one another during vacations or sick days.

The third option is day care. This is often a difficult hurdle to get over in terms of convincing your loved one to participate. He doesn't want to leave home. He doesn't want to spend his time with "those old people." He thinks he is being separated from you. (No, you can't convince him it is only during work hours when you aren't home anyway). I have heard of many excellent methods for getting past this resistance. You could tell him he's going to work or to volunteer at this place. You could tell him it's his social club, card club or that he's going out to lunch with friends. Invariably, the staff at the day care is more than willing to go along with this type of encouragement and give him tasks to do or ask his help in looking after the other participants or whatever it takes. Typically, once he gets past the first few days, he comes to enjoy 'his place.' I'm sure there are some exceptions, but I haven't heard of anyone who resisted or fought going, day after day, during the entire time they were participating. Day care is consistent, reliable and gives the employee-caregiver real peace of mind. You know your loved one is safe and secure, well fed and has company.

The fourth situation you will deal with is nursing home or assisted living care. While many people have difficulty envisioning this option, and feel guilty at the very thought of putting their loved one in a nursing home, rest assured that for a person with Alzheimer's, the nursing home environment can be beneficial. His primary need is consistency and routine in order function at his best. He needs a constant environment in order to make sense of his world. Statistically, the most difficult behaviors of an Alzheimer's patient disappear within a short time after moving to a nursing home. Following the same schedule with the same people day in and day out has a calming effect. Normally, we don't think of our homes as chaotic, but consider 'normal' life from the Alzheimer's person's point of view. You are in and out; your family is in and out; you have company; your kids have their friends coming by; the phone is ringing; you are taking him in the car to run to the store or do other errands; the mailman comes by; sales people may come to the door. There is a busy-ness about a normal household that can make a person with Alzheimer's dizzy. This is the most frequent reason he becomes agitated and/or withdrawn. A nursing home, particularly the one which knows dementia, is a calm, constant environment without too many 'surprises' that the individual has to try to process. But you have to do your homework.

You want to look at several nursing homes to get a feel for how they compare. Notice how well all the staff seems to know the residents. (Does the receptionist at the main desk say hello and call them by name? Does the maintenance staff seem comfortable around people with dementia?) Is the facility clean? If you are there during meal time, can you tell what food is being served by the smell, or is there a sort of generic, 'institutional food' smell? When you go for an appointment, how many staff members meet you? If it's only one, does he or she take you to the floor and interact with the other staff and residents?   If the only person you meet is an administrative person who doesn't seem to know the residents or floor staff, this is not a good sign. Are the residents clean and dressed? Do the mentally alert patients seem happy and congenial with one another?

Go to visit nursing homes without an appointment. If you know someone there, go to visit her and sit in a community room or near the nurses station with her. You can learn a lot by observing for a little while. While there, interact with some of the other residents. People in nursing homes almost always love to have company whether they know you or not.

Once the searching is over and you have placed your loved one in a nursing home, go to visit often. Get involved in your loved one's care. Let the nursing home staff know you are there to help and support them, not to get in the way and complain. Visit often and at different times and days. Even in the best of nursing homes, there is a tendency for the staff to be a little more attentive to the residents whose families come frequently and at unpredictable times. As you get to know each of the staff members, find out what they do really well and <u>tell them</u>. Nursing home staff work very hard, very long hours for very little pay and they need all the support and encouragement they can get. (And feed them. Nothing like cookies or brownies to earn points with the staff!)

If it seems like they don't see your loved one as you do, there's a reason. Consider the perspective they are coming from. They have met this person who already is well-advanced in Alzheimer's Disease. They have no idea what he was like before. And they accept him as he is with all the difficulties and limitations of his disease. They are building a relationship with him that isn't based on what could have been but rather on what is. Watch them. The best of aides and nurses will tune into your loved one like no one else you've seen. All your family and friends look at him with a touch of sadness. The nursing home staff will look at him with a practical, positive attitude that makes him feel accepted just as he is.

Finally, as a caregiver – employed or otherwise – seek out a support group for yourself. Whether you are in the first phases of experiencing this disease, or it's been going on for what seems like forever; whether you are caring for him at his home, in your home, long distance, or in a nursing home, seek out a support group. There are few things that will give you the energy to keep going like spending time with others who are or have been where you are. There is such encouragement in talking about shared experience. If the first one you try doesn't quite fit, try another. There are many different groups and each has a flavor of its own. Find one that suits your personality. Check with your local Alzheimer's Association, Hospice or Social Services organization. Oftentimes, nursing homes have their own family support groups.

Balancing the obligations of work and home care is not always easy, but if you make the effort to look for help, you will find it.

"I believe Alz. disease must be like going to a new job on the first day. I'm sure you can recall the many questions entering your mind as you approached that first day on the new job. Where is the bathroom? Where do I put my purse? When do I go to lunch? Where do I eat lunch? Who are all these people? Just imagine now how it must be for a person with dementia. Every day is like this."[1]

[1] Haisman, Pam RN. (1998). Alzheimer's Disease: Caregivers Speak Out, p 216. Chippendale House Publishers. Ft. Myers, FL

Chapter IX

Encouragement

Maureen Reagan died while I was in the process of writing this book. What a fine lady she was and a great advocate for Alzheimer's understanding and research. I had the privilege of meeting her at the World Alzheimer's Congress in Washington DC in July of 2000. I greeted her as a fan would greet a known personality. She responded as if we were friends. As I watched her that evening, she was gracious and friendly to everyone she spoke with. Her speech on behalf of Alzheimer's research was doubly moving because she clearly spoke from personal experience. You can tell fairly quickly whether a speaker is just talking about the topic of Alzheimer's or speaking from the vantage point of one who has walked with this disease. Ms. Reagan clearly fell into the latter category. It was obvious that she had spent a good deal of time with her Dad since his illness.

In all the speeches I have heard her give, while she never minimized the tragedy of Alzheimer's Disease, she always spoke of the bright moments with her father, of the things he could do rather than the things he couldn't do. You could feel the joy she gained from these 'golden moments.' During one speech, a gentleman in the audience got up and said that people always ask him why he keeps going to see his wife when she doesn't know who he is. His response was, "It doesn't matter. I know who she is." Ms. Reagan thanked him profusely for putting into words the reason we all, as caregivers, do what we do. We know who our loved ones are, who our residents, clients, and parishioners are. We know that we can give ourselves to them and make their lives worthwhile wherever they are in their journeys.

Did you ever have the experience of leaving a baby with a babysitter while you had to work? Did you feel as though you missed some of his most special moments; the learning moments that will only come once? These are golden moments, the fleeting, passing joys you miss if you're not there, paying attention, watching. Similarly, for the person with Alzheimer's, there are golden moments you will miss if you're not tuned in. I had a lovely lady tell me one day of her mother who no longer responded to her as daughter. This daughter was feeling pretty saddened by this but visited her mother frequently. One time, she had to go out of town for a funeral and was gone a few days. When she returned, she went right to the nursing home and as she walked into the dayroom, her mother threw open her arms and said, "My baby!!" That was a moment this daughter will cherish for the rest of her life, even if her mother never outwardly shows signs of recognition again.

Golden moments are seeing your mother rock and caress her baby doll and you know she's reliving her early motherhood; sharing a laugh over something you wouldn't have thought she realized was funny; having an aide tell you how she (non-verbally) scolded him, shaking her finger at him, for taking away her 'baby' when it was supper time; seeing a look of joy when a resident wins a little prize at a carnival; hearing a resident say upon being given a colorful, but complex, rod and bead puzzle, "Get this thing away from me. I'm crazy enough as it is."; hearing a resident spontaneously recite the Our Father and then ask, hopefully, "Did I get it right?"; seeing the visual response in a person at infancy level to the scent of a gardenia, a treasure from her past. There are so many golden moments occurring daily that make you glad for having waded through the difficulties. Don't miss them.

Have there been times when you have regretted things you have or haven't done for your loved one? Have you felt inadequate to the task of caregiving? I once read a book called <u>Your Best is Good Enough</u>, by Vivian Greenberg. It's written primarily to adult children caring for their parents, but the sentiments and encouragement are applicable to any caregiver. I read it several years ago, and it was of real benefit to me throughout my caregiving years. Even just contemplating the title phrase, 'your best is good enough,' should remind all of us that no one reaches the 'ideal' in caregiving; all we can aim for is our best. And that deserves applause. Applaud yourself if no one else is around to do it. At the end of each day, don't look back and regret the mistakes you made, but find the good you did and rejoice in that. I've talked to people who say, "But I'm so exhausted by the end of the day, I can't think of anything good that I did or that happened." Was it a calm day? You made it calm. If there were there upsets during the day, were they resolved? You succeeded in resolving them. Was the day one disaster after another? Well, maybe the one thing you accomplished was to get this person into bed and sleeping and that's a major hurdle. And think back, was the morning a good one before the 'trouble' started. Keep in mind, too, that tomorrow he won't remember that you upset him today. Maybe you just got him to eat a meal, or maybe you had a pleasant walk, or you made him laugh. Whatever went well this day – take credit for it.

Here's another positive aspect about Alzheimer's Disease. In the earlier stages of this disease, while the person is still talking, take advantage of his clarity with regard to the past and learn stories about his youth/childhood you might not have known. Encourage him to talk about who he was (or where he is now). Not only could it be interesting, but having someone ask questions and listen to his stories can build his self image and confidence as well.

What follows are passages that I found very encouraging from talks and writings of various people, some of whom have Alzheimer's and some of whom have witnessed it in their personal or professional lives.

"Sometimes I picture myself like a candle. I used to be a candle eight feet tall – burning bright. Now every day I lose a little bit of me. Someday the candle will be very small – but the flame will be just as bright." I came across this quotation on the Internet written by a woman with Alzheimer's. I was struck by the optimism expressed in the last phrase.

"The caregiver is meeting an infinitely demanding circumstance with a terribly finite resource – one's self. Life with the loved one can provide the gift of reversing that sensation; the disease is finite, and the caregiver is equipped with infinite resources.

"The human spirit is graced with an awesome capacity to embrace the most heinous of circumstances and to find there the realm of the sacred." (*Ewing, Wayne A. PhD, An Existential Dimension, a presentation for the World Alzheimer's Congress, July 2000, Washington DC. These observations are developed in Mr. Ewing's book, Tears In God's Bottle, AuthorHouse*)

"The phrase, the 'burden of caregiving' is used almost exclusively to describe the care of our elderly. Every time you use the word burden in relationship to caregiving, you are imprinting a negative image. Child rearing is a challenge; caregiving is a challenge. We have to stop denigrating the care of our elderly as being something out of the ordinary." (*Bigtree Murphy, Beverly MS,CRC, Twelve Things Not To Say To a Caregiver*)

"Every person has value apart from memory. Caregiving needn't be looked at only from the perspective of stress and adaptation to stress. It can be something more than a burden.

"Think of what good things you have gotten/learned from the experience. You're not going to get close to a person's spirit if you think in terms of management, care, or burden. If we can understand how to treat each person as a whole person, then we'll find most of the answers."

(*Bell, Virginia MSW, Bell, Rev. Wayne, Lexington KY, Touching the Human Spirit Through Quality Care, National Alzheimer's Conference, July 1998, Indianapolis, IN*)

"Our attention should shift from caregiver burden to caregiver gain. Gain is the extent to which the caregiving role is appraised to enhance an individual's life and be enriching." This author goes on to say that caregivers appraise their task not based on the demands or their relative's disturbances or lack of support, but rather on the sense of right or wrong or fairness of the task. Family members who appear the least stressed are those who see the caregiving task in terms of

- a commitment or opportunity (not obligation) to 'repay' loved one
- knowing he is getting proper care
- closeness to loved one
- opportunity to get to know him

- he deserves my best

(*Gesino, Jack Paul DSW, New Haven, CT, <u>Assessing Family Ethics</u>, World Alzheimer's Congress, July 2000, Washington DC*)

"I've noticed that I have a large amount of appreciation for whatever I'm focused on. It's very clear and real; a look away and it's gone. Look back and it's fresh and new. I am checking this out with a red geranium right now. When I look away, 'red' no longer exists except as an abstract term. No blossom image remains. But I can look again. . ." (*Internet message from Laura to Morris Friedell: both Alzheimer's victims*)

"In dementia, or other such catastrophes, however great the organic damage, there remains the undiminished possibility of reintegration by art, by communion, by touching the human spirit … A person does not consist of memory alone. He has feeling, will, sensibilities, moral being – matters of which neuro-psychology cannot speak." (reprinted with the permission of Simon & Schuster Adult Publishing Group from <u>The Man Who Mistook His Wife for a Hat and Other Clinical Tales</u> by Oliver Sacks. Copyright © 1970, 1981, 1984, 1985)

"I hear people say that Alzheimer's people lose their humanity. A lot is lost, but not that. Just last week, I went to see my mother, and she was sitting next to a woman who's completely nonverbal. My mother, who has never been that demonstrative, was holding this woman's hand and stroking her face. And I thought, 'How dare anyone say these people have lost their humanity!'

"A rather verbal resident who can no longer coordinate her speech with her mind, came into the room of another resident who was very ill and dying. She just sat by the bedside for an hour and stroked the ill resident's arm. Then, in a fully cognizant moment, she said, 'I don't think she is going to be with us much longer.' What insight! What recognition! So please don't ever underestimate what might be going on in the mind of a person with Alzheimer's. Often their hearts and heads are fully aware, even if their words or actions do not match." (*Haisman, Pam RN,MS, Alzheimer's Disease: Caregivers Speak Out, p 179, Chippendale House Publishers, Ft. Myers, FL, 1998*)

This next rather lengthy and moving quote is from an emergency room doctor who eloquently describes how our viewpoint can change when we pay attention, get up close and see the very soul before us.

"They lie there, breathing heavy gasps, contracted into a fetal position. Ironic, that they should live 80 or 90 years, then return to the posture of their childhood. But they do. Sometimes their voices are mumbles and whispers like those of infants or toddlers. I have seen them, unaware of anything for decades, crying out for parents long since passed away.

"Usually the feeling comes in those times when I am weary and frustrated from making too many decisions too fast, in the middle of the night. Into the midst of this comes a patient from a local nursing home, sent for reasons I can seldom discern.

"I walk into the room and roll my cynical eyes at the nurse. She hands me the minimal data sent with the patient, and I begin the detective work. And just when I'm most annoyed, just when I want to do nothing and send them back, I look at them. And then I touch them. And then, as I imagine my sons, tears well up and I see the error of my thoughts. For one day, it may be.

"One day, my little boys, still young enough to kiss me and think me heroic, may lie before another cynical doctor, in the middle of the night of their dementia, and need care. More than medicine, they will need compassion. They will need someone to have the insight to look at them and say, 'Here was once a child, cherished and loved, who played games in the nursery with his mother and father. Here was a child who put teeth under pillows, and loved bedtime stories, crayons and stuffed animals. Here was a treasure of love to a man and a woman long gone. How can I honor them? By treating their child with love and gentility. By seeing that their child has come full circle to infancy once more, and will soon be born once more into forever.'

"This vision is frightful because I will not be there to comfort them, or to say, "I am here" when they call out, unless God grants me the gift of speaking across forever. It is painful because I will not be there to serve them as I did in life, and see that they are treated as what they are: unique and wonderful, made in the image of the Creator, and of their mother and me. It is terrible because our society treats the aged as worse than a burden; it treats them as tragedies of time. It seems hopeless because when they contract and lie motionless, no one will touch them with the love I have for them, or know the history of their scars, visible and invisible. I am the walking library of their lives, and I will be unavailable.

"And yet, the image has beauty and hope as well. I can imagine that even if they live in their shadowland alone, somewhere children and grandchildren, even great-grandchildren thrive. I can hope that their heirs come to see them, and care, and harass the staff of the nursing home to treat Grandpa better. I can hope that they dare not allow my boys to suffer, but that they hold no illusions about physical immortality and will let them come to their mother and me when the time arrives. And best, I can know that their age and illness will only bring the day of that reunion closer.

"My career as an emergency physician has taught me something very important about dealing with the sick and injured, whether young or old. It has taught me that the Golden Rule also can be stated this way: 'Do unto others as you would have others do unto your children.' I think that this is a powerful way to improve our interactions with others, not just in medicine but in every action of our lives. And it is certainly a unique way to view our treatment of the elderly. For one day all our children will be old. And only if this lesson has been applied will they be treated with anything approaching the love that only we, their parents, hope for them to always have." (*Leap, Dr. Edwin, The Golden Rule Revisited, Emergency Medical News, Vol. 22, Issue 10, Oct. 2000, p.18*)

This quote is from a priest who wasn't involved with Alzheimer's, but some of the comments he made have such a profound meaning for caregivers as well as people who have Alzheimer's. Father Walter Ciszek, a Soviet prisoner in Siberia for 23 years, wrote that he spent much of his life trying to understand the will of God. He agonized over the fact that for much of his life, he was unable to carry out his priestly duties. Finally, it became clear to him that *the circumstances in which he found himself were God's will for him.*

"We had to learn to look at our daily lives, at everything that crossed our path each day, with the eyes of God; learning to see His estimate of things, places, and above all, people, recognizing that He had a goal and a purpose in bringing us into contact with these things and these people, and striving always to do that will – His will – every hour of every day in the situations in which He had placed us."

Then he wrote "…that every moment of our life has a purpose, that every action of ours has a dignity and a worth beyond human understanding. No man's life is insignificant in God's sight, nor are his works insignificant. Yet what a responsibility is here. For it means that no moment can be wasted, no opportunity missed, since each has a purpose in man's life, each has a purpose in God's plan." (*Ciszek, Fr. Walter SJ, He Leadeth Me,pp 38, 201 Ignatius Press, SanFrancisco, CA, 1973*)

"Time passes and does not return. God has assigned to each of us a definite time in which to fulfill His divine plan for our soul; we have only this time and shall have no more. Our life is made up of this uninterrupted, continual flow of time, which never returns." (*Fr. Gabriel of St. Mary Magdalen, O.C.D., Divine Intimacy, p 103, Tan Books and Publishers, Rockford, IL, 1964*)

Whether you are a caregiver of a loved one, a professional caregiver, police officer or emergency worker, a research scientist or someone in the medical field, a minister or just someone who encounters the Alzheimer's person in a brief interaction, remember that every moment has a purpose in God's plan.

POSTSCRIPT

An expression which I find rather troublesome is 'quality of life.' Often, it is used by those who are in good health when making certain assumptions about those who are not. It becomes a very subjective concept, disassociated with real life: I may be 25, 30, 50 years younger than the person in question, but I decide he has a poor quality of life because he cannot do the things that I think he should enjoy. I may even apply it to myself. Perhaps at age 40 I tell family and friends, if I reach the point where I cannot travel or participate in a particular activity or sport, I won't have a decent quality of life and, therefore, want my life ended. The problem is that no one can speak for another, nor can we project our needs and wants into the future. More importantly, we have no right to deliberately end life, our own or anyone else's.

As we age, our interests and comfort level changes. We may come to prefer more family time and less travel, and different or more sedentary activities, and may very well be quite content. What may seem to be a rather sad or humdrum life to a 17 year old is probably just fine for a 90 year old.

On the other hand, I do believe in the 'value of life.' All life has value and purpose. Whether it be to our own benefit or to someone else's, there is a purpose. I believe God has a plan for each one of us and each of these individual plans fit into a larger 'Master plan.' We may or may not know during our lifetime what our specific role or purpose is in that master plan. It is possible this purpose is not something we do in and of ourselves but rather how our being affects someone else. So, God puts us down on our particular path and we set off toward our goal (eternity, Heaven). On the way, we encounter a multitude of environments, circumstances and events, and many people cross our paths. Our objective, whether we know our purpose or not, is to follow this path the best we can, interacting faithfully with the circumstances and people whose paths cross ours, always keeping our eye on the goal which is God Himself. If we stray off our given path, we move farther and farther from the goal. How do we know when we've strayed? When we convince ourselves that life should be a bed of roses, total comfort, ease and fun. Real life, in fact, consists of comfort and discomfort; ease and disease; fun and sadness.

If we do everything in our power to avoid the pains and sorrows of life, we are off the path. We think, "I shouldn't have to suffer like this." (Why not?) Or, "My loved one shouldn't have to suffer." (But this is real life, remember?) If we think this way, the next logical step is to eliminate the person, and, therefore, eliminate his pain. As a convenient coincidence, we eliminate our own pain, suffering, inconvenience. We no longer need to care, to sacrifice our time and emotions for him, nor do we have the responsibility to hurt because he is hurting. What else do we get rid of in the process? The chance to grow, to become caring, to be there and to feel for and with another human being. What a terrible loss that would be. "And the King will answer them, 'Truly, I say to you, as you did it to one of the least of these my brethren, you did it to Me.'" (Mt 25:40) Should we risk missing the opportunity to serve God Himself?

I hope, in reading this book, you were able to put aside thoughts such as "This is terrible." or "No one should have to bear this." This is life. This is reality. This is real life. Jump into it with both feet. It always fascinates me when I hear people say they can't 'bear' something. Typically, they are not the ones who are required to 'bear' the thing. "Oh, I just can't bear to go see John in the nursing home. I can't bear to see him someplace other than in his own home." Well, he has to bear it doesn't he? "I can't bear to go to the funeral for that child who died. It's just too sad." But then, the family has to bear it don't they? We have to step out of ourselves and go where the other is. Walking our own path means suffering sometimes – suffering ourselves, or helping another through his or her suffering.

Henry Bugbee, a philosopher, used an expression that I believe speaks volumes. "Enduring is truer than withholding." We may not be in a caregiving or caring role by choice or with enthusiasm, but to endure with and for the person afflicted with Alzheimer's Disease brings untold benefits. I lived through almost 15 years of my mother's disease and would never have chosen that path for her or for myself, but as time went on … and on … and on … it became a way of life, to the point where I was a bit puzzled when people expressed sadness or sympathy on my behalf. They were kind, but I didn't feel my 'normal' life warranted pity. Now that it is over, I am overwhelmed by the blessings and benefits that came with it. The things I learned, the friends I made, the people in her life who became better caregivers for having known her: Mom's particular path crossed with many others whose journeys were enhanced for having known her. And for those of us who were blessed to witness it, we are grateful for her life.

If a person has been diagnosed as terminal, whatever disease or condition he has is leading to his death. I don't believe we can introduce another element that will hurry that process along. To say, "Well, they're dying anyway," is not just cause to circumvent the natural process. Fr. Frank Pavone (Priests For Life) made this comment with regard to the issues of euthanasia and suicide, "I'd hate to think of rushing into the presence of God uninvited." God's got the plan all worked out. We can only do our best to correspond to that plan.

Finally, I offer you this prayer by Cardinal John Henry Newman:

God has created me to do Him some definite service: He has committed some work to me which He has not committed to another.

I have my mission – I may never know it in this life, but I shall be told of it in the next.   I am a link in a chain, a bond of connection between persons.   He has not created me for naught.   I shall do good.   I shall do His work.   I shall be an angel of peace, a preacher of truth in my own place, while not intending it, if I do but keep His commandments.   Therefore, I will trust Him.   Whatever, wherever I am, I can never be thrown away.   If I am in sickness, my sickness may serve Him; in perplexity, my perplexity may serve Him; if I am in sorrow, my sorrow may serve Him.

He does nothing in vain.   He knows what He is about.   He may take away my friends; He may throw me among strangers.   He may make me feel desolate, make my spirits sink, hide my future from me.   Still, He knows what He is about."

APPENDIX A

Communication and Care

Each of the following statements describes the type of things you should find out about a person's past life by questioning him and/or his family. Given this information, what would you expect from these residents? What could you offer them to put them at ease?

1. *Al was a military officer. Subsequent to his career in the service, he became the Director of a local service agency and sat on the Board of Directors of a local sports team. He had three children and six grandchildren and an excellent sense of humor.*

Used to having control, giving orders, being listened to, this gentleman will require that you show him extra respect. Call him by his former title (Col., Lt., etc.) or 'sir.' Allow him as much control over his daily decisions as possible. Encourage him to help plan or supervise activities. He would have family interests, enjoy groups and laughter. Encourage the family to bring pictures. Talk with him about those family pictures often. Include him in mature group activities. Talk to him about travel; ask where he's been, what he's seen. You can take any positive information he provides and relate it back to him on days when he can't recall happier and prouder memories on his own.

2. *Barb was a secretary, single, and happily solitary in her lifestyle. She had two cats and enjoyed gardening. She was always very particular about her home and appearance, needing to have things 'just so.'*

This is a woman who will probably be quiet, gentle, neat and particular about her room and possessions. She is contented to be alone. She will be stressed by wanderers and by crowds. Approach her with a quiet manner. Do not force her into large group activities, but offer such things as movies or gardening activities. Provide picture books of cats or flowers. Be proactive in keeping wanderers out of her room. Allow her to help straighten things in the family or dining rooms of the facility.

3. *Frank was a university professor, an avid reader and patron of the local philharmonic orchestra. He is a musician and speaks several languages. He most often dressed in a proper, if not formal, manner – didn't even own a pair of jeans. He had no interest in sports, but always sought intellectually stimulating events.*

This gentleman will probably be a loner and prefer to remain in his room. He will be most comfortable dressing more formally. Do not force group activities, however, he may be pleased if he is asked to play music for others. Provide him with classical music. When he can no longer read, try books on tape. Allow him to dress as he wishes and be proactive in keeping wanderers out of his room. If any staff members or volunteers speak a foreign language, give him the opportunity to use his language skills with them.

4. Helen was a physical education teacher. She and her husband were great sports enthusiasts. They played golf or tennis whenever they got the chance and owned season tickets for the local hockey and baseball games.

This individual will be outgoing and physically active. She enjoys group activities, especially physically challenging ones. She may be (unintentionally) too aggressive with other residents. Enlist her help in moving tables and chairs around for activities, physical housekeeping chores. Allow her to take the lead in activities, but supervise closely if she is around more frail residents. Talk to her about sports, past and present. Who are her favorite teams? What types of games did she like to play or watch?

5. Henry was a European immigrant. He fought during World War II, lost his family and home and was a POW during the last several months of the war. Since coming to America, he has had a tailoring shop. He talked very little to people partly because of his accent, and partly because he was very reserved and withdrawn.

He may initially come across as a very strong, self-sufficient person or as very fearful and withdrawn, but is an emotionally frail person. Nervous and anxious about sudden moves and aggressive physical care, he needs to be cared for gently, slowly and with calming conversation. He may be mistrustful, and also may not make his wishes known. Be cautious about who cares for this resident. A person can, for no apparent reason, trigger bad memories for this man, and a change of caregivers should be made. Work with him slowly to determine what and with whom he is comfortable. If he trusts you, ask him about his experience during the war. Reassure him frequently that he is safe and cared for. Have family or friends provide tapes in his native language. If he is able, give him mending tasks to do.

In the following incidents, try to determine what need the individual trying to fill; to express themselves, to feel loved/secure, or to feel productive or useful? How would you handle these behaviors?

1. *A resident takes linens, gets into closets, bathrooms; tries to clean tables.*

Clearly, this person needs to be useful. By all means, allow him to fix, clean, fold, etc.

2. *Resident wants to 'go home.'*

This person is looking for some type of security. Chances are, home isn't the house he most recently came from. Ask about his home. Where is it; what color is it; what did you do there; who will be there; what will we do when we go there? He is looking for the security of his past. If you ask the right question, you may be able to fill that need with warm memories.

3. *A resident sitting in the hall calls out to each one passing by: "Help me." or "I'm hungry." or "Have you seen _____?", anything to get attention.*

He probably has a need to express himself and be heard. Stop and talk to him every little while. Put him near another resident who will listen to him. Remember that the need for attention is a legitimate need.

4. *Resident says, "My Mother just died."*

This person may be feeling a need for love or just looking for an avenue to express himself. Express sympathy and ask about his relationship with his mother. Don't try reality; i.e. 'You're 90 years old. Your mother died years ago.' That won't make any sense to the person and may get him more agitated. He knows how he feels. Empathize with that.

5. *A resident is struggling to get up and out of his chair.*

This fellow is looking to be productive or useful and this plays out in his need to go somewhere. If you have the time, and he is able, get him up and walk him for a bit, and do this for him every little while. Then on returning him to his chair – or another chair – provide something for him to read or do or fix.

APPENDIX B

Police Encounters

1. *You're working nights. At 2:00 in the morning, you see an elderly person walking down the street by himself. When you stop to question him, he is somewhat vague, but insistent that he has to go to work. What do you do?*

This man has probably woken out of a sound sleep and has it in his mind that it's time to get up and go to work. Because of his intense focus and inability to interpret his environment, the fact that it's dark or cold doesn't mean anything to him. Logic will not work here.

Look for Safe Return or hospital bracelet before doing anything else.

Try to 'go where he is' by asking about his work (or his destination). This will reassure him and cause him to turn his focus to you. Ask him where he works; what he does. Comment on that and encourage him to tell you more. When he realizes that you aren't exactly stopping him, and as he turns his attention to you, he should also become a little more alert through conversing. Now look for identification. Ask him what his name is and if he knows his address. (Caution: he may give you a childhood address). Does he have a wallet? Check his clothing for name labels.

Depending on what his work is, try to derail him and convince him that he can go in later. "Meanwhile, suppose I take you home and we'll get a cup of coffee while we wait." Usually by the time you get him home, he will have forgotten what his intent was. (Say he's trying to get to a store. Drive by a closed store and tell him, "Oh well, the store is closed. Supposing I take you home and you can come back later when it's open.")

If you can't get an address, or he gives a wrong address, drive around nearby streets to see if someone is looking for him. Chances are, if he's on foot, he hasn't gotten too far from his home and he may recognize it, or a neighbor may recognize him. You could also inquire at a nearby convenience store or Church whether they have ever seen this person before. Otherwise take typical missing person steps.

2. *You get called to a family trouble. When you arrive, a woman answers the door and she is crying and distraught. She tells you her husband has Alzheimer's and she is at the end of her rope. She can't handle it any more and wants you to do something. What do you do?*

First of all, if it appears that the husband is in no immediate danger or difficulty, try to get the woman aside, outside or in another room (but make sure you can see the husband in case he decides to wander off). Find out if she has any local family or other supportive friends she can call or whom you can call for her. If she doesn't and truly seems to be all alone in this situation, get her to talk to you about the situation. She may have been handling this by herself for a very long time with no one to talk to. (Caregivers tend to become isolated). There's a possibility that all she needs at this moment in time is a sounding board – that's you.

Next recommend she call the Alzheimer's Association. In fact, encourage her to do that right while you are there. They can offer help and assistance, refer her to other respite organizations (in home respite care and nursing homes that provide respite options), a listing of day care centers, and provide her with a list of support groups. If she has been isolated for a period of time, just finding out that these options are available can be a relief.

If she does have family or supportive friends, contact them to come and relieve her for a while. Suggest she might go by herself to see some day care centers.

If the husband is violent, take steps as listed in Chapters IV and VII. Try to determine from the wife what sets him off and what are his comforts. Try to remove him from the immediate environment, to another room perhaps or outside. Walk him down the street. If he is speaking clearly, question whatever he is talking about or just validate what he is feeling. For instance, if he says (yells), "She's trying to keep me trapped in that house!" you might respond, "That must be very frustrating." Then when he agrees with that, you might try something like, "Maybe she needs you there to protect her. Maybe she doesn't want to be alone." This type of response may appeal to his need to feel control in his life. He now has a reason to decide for himself that he will stay home.

Whatever the cause of his anger, don't just tell him to calm down. Tell him you're sure this must make him very angry and ask him to tell you more about it. He should calm down just by being able to express himself to someone who seems to understand.

The husband may just be anxious and restless. His wife's tension increases his own. Try calming measures. Get him alone, speak quietly, find out where he is and go there. If you can't get him to tell you anything, take him around the house and ask about pictures or other items in the house. This should change his focus. If the wife is hovering, ask her if she could make coffee or get you some water.

Your primary focus should be to calm the atmosphere in the home and then make suggestions for the wife to get assistance. She may not even know what her needs are, but if she follows up on your suggestions, others can help her to distance herself from the day to day stress. It may be as simple a matter as letting her talk to you. If she has had no outside influences for a long time, she will probably come away from the event telling everyone how very helpful you were. You don't have to solve their problems. You only have to recognize what they are and validate that they are legitimate.

3. *You stop a somewhat erratic driver. His rate of speed keeps changing and he appears not to know where he is going. When you approach him, he laughs and says something like, "It's the darndest thing. I thought I knew where the hardware store was, but I can't seem to find it. I'm okay, just a little forgetful today is all." What do you do?*

First of all, don't just direct him to the nearest hardware store and send him on his way. If he is indeed looking for a neighborhood location, it's not normal to forget where it is. Ask him if he just came from home and if he can tell you what his address is. Suggest that you follow him home or drive him home to see that he gets there all right.

Determine if there are other family members living with him and discuss the situation with them. This may be one of the earliest signs of Alzheimer's that has manifested itself, and the family may not even know. People with Alzheimer's are very good at hiding symptoms at the beginning. Suggest that they take steps to get a diagnosis.

If they do know there is a problem, suggest to them that he shouldn't be driving. They may be in agreement, but haven't been able to take the keys away as yet. As an authority figure, you may be the answer to their dilemma. Tell him that because of the unsafe driving you observed earlier, he cannot drive until he takes a driving test. He may accept that from you where he would never do so from a daughter, son or wife.

You may get one of two reactions. He will either be very angry with you for having brought him home and questioned his family, or he will be relieved for the help and glad that you've talked to his family. This will depend on where he is in terms of needing to deny this illness or needing the security of supervision. The anger is purely, "I don't know what's wrong with me and I can't deal with someone making me face it." The relief comes from a similar feeling. "I don't know what's wrong with me, but thank goodness someone is taking charge of things."

Research indicates that the symptoms of memory loss, disorientation and changes in spatial perception may result in drivers becoming lost, misjudging distances, forgetting basic rules of the road, becoming easily frustrated or having slower and incorrect reactions when making the multiple quick decisions needed to drive safely. Despite these facts, it is very difficult for some people to recognize the impact of the disease on their driving performance.

4. *You are called to take a report on a missing person. When you arrive, you are told that the missing person has dementia. How do you proceed?*

First, inquire if the person is registered with Safe Return. If so, contact that agency so they can fax that person's information and photo to nearby police agencies. If not, recommend that the family register for it as soon as possible.

Then you would proceed as with any missing person incident. However, in addition to the routine questions, ask whether the individual has ever wandered before and where did he go previously. Find out if there is any particular place he has gone with any frequency – a store, Church, club, etc. It's possible he may have gone to a familiar place but couldn't find his way back. Had he been talking about work or a house or anything from his past that he may be looking for?

Take something familiar of his with you so that when you find him, he'll feel a sense of security and come with you. If it's cold, bring his coat since it is very likely he wandered off without it. When you find him, approach him using the techniques listed in Chapters III and VII.

5. *A person reports a crime has taken place (robbery, assault). As you question the victim, you become aware that he has dementia. How do you proceed?*

In these cases, you are dealing with one of three things. Either he is delusional and the whole incident is imaginary, or it's based in reality, but happened perhaps 50 years ago, or it really occurred as he describes. This is probably one of the hardest situations to sort out.

Never automatically assume the report is not true, even though in the majority of cases it probably isn't. If it's a physical crime against the person, there should be evidence of that. If it's an accusation of theft, it's a lot less concrete. Chances are, the person will not be alone or there may be family or friends with whom you can get in contact. Question them about the incident. They may be able to provide information as to whether this person has imagined this type of thing in the past, or if this is, in fact, something that happened to them many years previously. Remember that the individual may be living that past very vividly.

Typically, if it is his imagination, he will be angry, but not necessarily frightened or anxious. If you determine this to be the case, go through the motions of filling out a report and reassure him you will follow up. This may be all he needs to calm down, having someone take him seriously.

If he is frightened or extremely anxious, it may be a real incident. If it occurred years ago, there really isn't much you can do but sympathize, encourage him to tell you about it and try to redirect him onto another subject. It may relieve his anxiety if you 'take a report.' If it is a real incident, locate a family member or friend/neighbor to assist the person and proceed as you would with any criminal incident.

Note: If you have any reason to believe the person is being taken advantage of by relatives or acquaintances, get in touch with Social Services. Abuse of the elderly, especially those with dementia, is far too frequent and very easy to hide.

APPENDIX C

<u>Emergency Room Situations</u>

Frequently, patients are brought into the emergency room from assisted living facilities or skilled nursing facilities with no family member or caregiver to assist them. The following situations assume that a caregiver is not present and staff needs to facilitate the treatment without any input from one who knows the patient.

1. *A patient is brought in for a minor injury or illness. The ER is extremely busy, and typically, minor injuries are given lower priority. These patients can wait. However, this person, while not anxious or aggressive, becomes increasingly restless.*

The person with Alzheimer's does not understand why he is waiting, why he is in a strange place, nor will explanations do any good. Unless he is a fairly quiet individual (or falls asleep), he will become restless pretty quickly, and attempt to leave. Or he may just wander around and get into things he shouldn't. In so far as is possible, given the hectic environment of an emergency room, attend to him as soon as possible. Try not to make him wait. Also, whether it is a short or long wait, a dementia patient needs to have someone with him at all times. Provide him with something to do – looking at magazines will only last a matter of minutes – or get someone to push him around in a wheelchair while he is waiting. Just being able to move around will probably keep him somewhat contented. It's a lot easier to control him by wheeling him than by trying to keep him in one place.

2. *An ER staff member approaches the individual to perform whatever treatment is necessary and encounters resistance and/or fear.*

Keep in mind that no matter how advanced a person is in this disease, he maintains a normal emotional response. He will be very aware of your emotional presence and will react to it. In an emergency room situation, where he is already anxious because of the foreign environment, you must approach him in such a way that you don't appear to be in a hurry (even if you are). Don't have more than one or two people in the room with him. Call him by name and speak to him as if you already know him. Sit down and chat with him for a few minutes to reassure him that you are a friend. Even though you think you may not have time to do this, it may very well save you a good deal of time in the long run if you don't have to fight him to do your exam.

If he seems to have some level of understanding, try to explain why he is in the ER. If it's possible, allow him to sit up rather than lie down. Then, as you begin your exam or treatment, go slowly and tell him everything you are doing. Show him the instruments or supplies you are using, and perhaps, have him hold things for you while you carry out the procedure. If he is unable to communicate with, understand or assist you, use a calm, unhurried, reassuring tone and manner. Usually, Alzheimer's patients are very trusting and if you don't convey abruptness or a hurried manner, he should respond fairly well.

3. *A man with dementia is brought in and you are told he might become aggressive.*

Ideally, put him in a somewhat quiet room or area where he cannot see all the activities going on in the ER. All the incoming stimuli will be very difficult for him to process and could set off a chain reaction of confusion, fear, anger and aggression. Have a calm person sit and talk to him until it is time to treat him. You are trying to forestall any environmental triggers to his aggression. Triggers could be anything such as being in a strange place, extraneous sounds and activities, or no familiar faces.

As with the restless person, if he starts to become very anxious while waiting, get a wheelchair and take him for a walk down the hall for a bit. When it comes time to treat him, ask for his help. One of the things that will frequently set off a person is a sense of loss of control. If you give him the feeling that he is helping and making some decisions with you, he may be calmer. As noted in Chapter VII, move slowly and deliberately, explaining as you go along. If you start doing things in rapid sequence, he won't be able to process one thought or action before you have moved on to something else.

If, in spite of your efforts, he becomes combative, have one person hold his attention while others move people and objects out of harm's way. Try bringing in diversionary items – food, toys, cards, music. Consider that the one person with him may be causing the anger. There may be some unknown reason why he objects to him or her. Try bringing someone else into the picture. Sometimes a sudden firm voice will break the cycle. "John, what can I do for you?!" or "Here! Hold this!" or "What do you want?!"

When all else fails, obviously medical intervention will be needed, however, it is hoped that you can get his cooperation by trying to understand what his reality is and responding to that.

APPENDIX D

Clergy / Ministerial Situations

1. Suppose you have someone to visit in a skilled nursing facility. The staff doesn't know the individual's faith history. How do you find out if he had a religious background and what it was?

First, check around the room. There are usually clues there as to who this person is. Is there a cross or crucifix or holy pictures on the wall? A crucifix or pictures of Mary, for instance, would tell you he is Catholic. A cross or other types of holy pictures indicate that he may be Protestant. Look for greeting cards and see if any are signed by some clergy member or congregation. Take a look at family photos for clues. If there is absolutely nothing around the room to suggest a religious affiliation, start with the basics and see if you get a reaction from the resident. A positive reaction will tell you he is hearing something familiar. Try the Our Father, the Hail Mary or the 23rd Psalm. If none of these elicit a response, your best bet is to read familiar passages from the Old Testament which all faiths will be comfortable with. Even if he has had no religious background, he will probably enjoy having someone read to him.

2. What if you start to pray and the individual starts to holler?

If this person is fairly advanced in this disease and not able to communicate with words, he may, in his own way, be trying to join you. Notice if his expression calm or agitated. Does he stop when you stop? If he is trying to pray with you, he will probably listen for a little while when you start to pray again before he 'joins in.'

On the other hand, is his expression angry? If so, try playing hymns and see if you get the same reaction. He may find music more soothing.

If the person is still somewhat verbal and objects to your praying, stop and ask him why. Or ask him what he thinks about God. You may be able to carry on a brief conversation about God from his perspective and reaffirm him in whatever positive beliefs he has.

3. *You are ministering to an early stage Alzheimer's person and he tells you he wants to end his life. What do you do?*

If you tell him he's wrong and that he can't do this, he won't feel able to express his true feelings, right or wrong. Since he is speaking to you as a spiritual guide, he is probably looking for help in facing those feelings and wants to hear reasons why he shouldn't do this. You just want to help him come to that conclusion.

Acknowledge the validity of his feelings and reframe his statement. He says, "I want to die." You say, "You mean you don't want to be here any more?" Get him to express his thoughts as best he can and then gradually lead him around to the reasons he might not want to end his life – his family, friends, their true desire to care for him. Wouldn't he want to care for them if the situation were reversed? Let him know that he won't feel this way forever.

When you think he is ready for it, bring him to the spiritual aspects. God loves him and he has a plan for his life. This is just a part of that plan. We have to trust that God knows where that plan will lead, even if we don't. Reassure him that there will always be others, yourself included, who will pray for and with him, who will remember for him, and keep him spiritually connected.

SELECTED BIBLIOGRAPHY

Andresen, Gayle. <u>Caring for People With Alzheimer's Disease</u>. Health Professions Press. 1995.

Bell, Virginia; Troxel, David. <u>The Best Friends Approach to Alzheimer's Care</u>. Health Professions Press. 1996.

Brackey, Jolene. <u>Creating Moments of Joy</u>. Enhanced Moments. 1999.

Bugbee, Henry. <u>The Inward Morning</u>. University of Georgia Press. 1958.

*Ciszek, Fr. Walter. <u>With God In Russia</u>. 1964. <u>HeLeadeth Me</u>. 1973. Ignatius Press.

*Davis, Robert. <u>My Journey Into Alzheimer's Disease</u>. Tyndale House Publishers, Inc. 1989.

*DeBaggio, Thomas. <u>Losing My Mind</u>. 2002. <u>When It Gets Dark</u>. 2003. The Free Press.

Ewing, Wayne A. <u>Tears In God's Bottle: Reflections on Alzheimer's Caregiving</u>. Author House.

Graf, Peter; Ohta, Nobuo. <u>Lifespan Development of Human Memory</u>. MIT Press. 2002.

Grant, Linda. <u>Remind Me Who I Am Again</u>. Granta Publications. 1998.

Haisman, Pam. <u>Alzheimer's Disease: Caregivers Speak Out</u>. Chippendale House Publishers. 1998.

Henderson, Cary Smith. <u>Partial View: An Alzheimer's Journal</u>. SMU Press. 1998.

*Keck, David. <u>Forgetting Whose We Are</u>. Abingdon Press. 1996.

Mace, Nancy; Rabins, Peter. <u>The 36-Hour Day</u>. Warner Books. 1981.

McGowin, Diana Friel. <u>Living In the Labyrinth</u>. Elder Books. 1993.

McKim, Donald, ed. <u>God Never Forgets</u>. Westminster John Knox Press. 1997.

Medina, John. <u>What You Need to Know About Alzheimer's</u>. New Harbinger Publications. 1999.

<u>Research and Practice in Alzheimer's Disease,</u> Vol. 3. Springer Publishing Company. 2000.

Robinson, Anne; Spencer, Beth; White, Laurie. <u>Understanding Difficult Behaviors</u>. East Michigan University. 1989.

Sacks, Oliver. <u>The Man Who Mistook His Wife For a Hat and Other Clinical Tales</u>. Simon & Shuster Adult Publishing Group. 1985.

*Shenk, David. <u>The Forgetting</u>. Doubleday. 2001.

*Snowdon, David. <u>Aging With Grace</u>. Bantam Books. 2001.

Snyder, Lisa. <u>Speaking Our Minds</u>. W.H. Freeman and Company. 1999.

Strauss, Claudia. <u>Talking to Alzheimer's</u>. New Harbinger Publications, Inc. 2001.

*Tanzi, Rudolph; Parson, Ann. <u>Decoding Darkness</u>. Perseus Publishing. 2000.

Young, Ellen. <u>Between Two Worlds</u>. Prometheus Books. 1999.

*While I found all of these resources very beneficial, these I've marked are my personal favorites.

ABOUT THE AUTHOR

Born in 1947 in Rochester, NY, Patricia M. Thompson still resides there with her husband, Gary. They have four children: son, David and his wife Kelly, and daughter, Michelle, and her husband, Andrew. After raising her family, Patricia returned to college and obtained a bachelor's degree in Chemistry from SUNY Brockport. She worked in chemistry for several years, but over time, as three family members were diagnosed with Alzheimer's Disease, her interests turned in a different direction. Through various conferences, course work, and personal experience, she became proficient in the communication skills that are most effective in dealing with folks who have this disease. Besides caring for her own family members, she has been a volunteer with Hospice since 1986 and spends the majority of her volunteer time in nursing homes, frequently with Alzheimer's patients and their families. In 2000, she formed St. Colman Consulting, through which she offers presentations to police, clergy, nursing home staff, hospice personnel, as well as family groups and others. This book is the culmination of her work in the field of Alzheimer's.

Copies may be purchased from: www.lulu.com

The author may be reached at pmtscp@rochester.rr.com

myoclonal jerking, *13*